"*Help Me Live* is a deeply moving exploration of the complex range of emotions that arise in the face of illness. Both patients and caregivers can enter into their roles with greater acceptance and love from reading the experiences and interviews by Lori Hope. Lori's lists of ways to act, words to say give us the confidence to enter these sensitive arenas of vulnerability and fear with greater knowledge consciousness and confidence."

—Susan Halpern, MSW, author of *Etiquette of Illness*

"When people we love have cancer, we want to help them, but may not know how. *Help Me Live* puts you in direct contact with the true experts—people who have been through it, and offers you the opportunity to learn to support a cancer patient with compassion and intelligence. An insightful and very useful book."

—Martin L. Rossman, MD, author of *Fighting Cancer from Within*

"As a two-time survivor of breast cancer and a journalist, I found *Help Me Live* to be informative, touching, and even funny—and when it comes to cancer, you need a sense of humor. The author also certainly lives up to her name: Her own personal story of cancer and the stories of others give you *hope*. The book provides a valuable service of what you should and shouldn't say to cancer patients."

—Laura Marquez, ABC News correspondent

"Every family touched by cancer should read this book. Too often, people who have cancer are seen more as bearers of the disease than as who they actually are. That can leave them feeling isolated, hurt, and angry. Lori Hope's *Help Me Live* addresses this phenomenon with suggestions that are wise, clear, effective, and compassionate to all concerned."

—Jeff Kane, MD, Sierra Nevada Cancer Center,
author of *How to Heal: A Guide for Caregivers*

"*Help Me Live* is realistic but upbeat. Drawing on her experience, those of many others with cancer, and that of a number of leading health professionals, Lori provides sensible and sensitive guidelines for helping those with cancer and their families to live better. If you or a loved one is struggling with cancer, don't be without Hope."

—David Spiegel, MD, Stanford University, author of *Living Beyond Limits*

"If I could have given copies of the book to my friends and family, it would have saved me countless tense and unhappy moments."

—Karin Roosa, breast cancer survivor

"Lori Hope's masterful storytelling and clear explanations are invaluable for cancer survivors, helping you understand (and forgive) others' hurtful words and actions, and encouraging you to direct family and friends to responses that help. This book is a gift for caregivers and everyone who knows someone who is going through illness, helping you understand what helps or hurts (and why), but most important of all, showing you how to listen and care in healing ways."

—Wendy S. Harpham, MD, author of *Happiness in a Storm* and *Diagnosis: Cancer*

"What a remarkable book—patients with cancer often say to me, 'It's bad enough to have cancer, but would you BELIEVE what someone said to me the other day?' Those expressions are often not easily forgotten, when they caused either pain or joy. I really like Lori's use of these common expressions as the base for suggesting good etiquette and kind manners in talking to someone who has a serious illness."

—Jimmie Holland, MD, Memorial Sloan-Kettering Cancer Center, author of *The Human Side of Cancer*

"Filled with warmth, humor, compassion and love, Lori Hope guides us through her own experience with cancer and those of the individuals she interviewed. The advice, comments and suggestions contained within *Help Me Live* are meaningful and valuable to cancer patients, their families, friends, caregivers, physicians, and therapists as well as any compassionate individual living in a society with other human beings. Lori's hopeful and melodic voice sings throughout."

—Jo Ellen Lezotte, past president of The Cancer League, Inc.

"With grace and good humor, Hope tells us what we all should know about facing this life-altering disease. Extraordinarily moving and helpful, this book is essential reading for cancer patients as well as their families and friends."

—Marc Silver, author of *Breast Cancer Husband* and editor at *U.S. News & World Report*

help me live

help me live

20 things
people with cancer
want you to know

Lori Hope

CELESTIAL ARTS
Berkeley | Toronto

Celestial Arts
Box 7123
Berkeley, California 94707
www.tenspeed.com

Distributed in Australia by Simon and Schuster Australia, in Canada by Ten Speed
Press Canada, in New Zealand by Southern Publishers Group, in South Africa by
Real Books, and in the United Kingdom and Europe by Airlift Book Company.

Cover and text design by Nancy Austin

A portion of the proceeds from this book will be donated to organizations that
support people who have received a cancer diagnosis and those who care for them.

Quotes on pages 7 and 180 are copyright © 2005 Ashleigh Brilliant,
http://www.ashleighbrilliant.com.

Library of Congress Cataloging-in-Publication Data
Hope, Lori.
   Help me live : 20 things people with cancer want you to know / by
   Lori Hope.
      p. cm.
   Includes bibliographical references and index.
   ISBN-10: 1-58761-212-7 (pbk.)
   ISBN-13: 978-1-58761-212-1 (pbk.)
   1. Cancer—Popular works. 2. Cancer—Psychological
   aspects. I. Title.

RC263.H67 2005
616.99'4—dc22   2005008395

Printed in United States of America
First printing, 2005
1 2 3 4 5 6 7 8 9 10 — 09 08 07 06 05

*For David, of course,
and those who gave me life,
helped me live,
and shared their stories*

contents

acknowledgments

There are only two ways to live your life. One is as though nothing is a miracle. The other is as though everything is a miracle.

—Albert Einstein

Thank you for helping me live

One year ago, I was not sure I would survive the stab of the scalpel I had invited into my flesh. It was not the surgeon I mistrusted; it was life itself. About to undergo an operation to remove a tumor that I feared had fired microscopic missiles throughout my body, I had taken care of my most important affairs. When I silently mouthed, "Good-bye" to my loved ones in the softly lit presurgery room at sunrise, it felt like a final farewell.

How intoxicating to think that fifty-two weeks later, I not only breathe, but I am birthing a book about life. It is a book inspired by and dedicated to all those who have helped me live.

Thank you first to David, my best friend and husband, whose strength, faith, compassion, and of course love helped keep my heart beating always, and whose generosity and support enabled me to take the time I needed to explore this difficult subject; and to Brett, the best son ever, who helped ensure my survival by lovingly creating my "Caring Page" website, as well as by ridding our home of pestilence (we were visited not only by cancer, but by ants and raccoons last summer).

Thank you to Dad, Mamma Jude, RSASJ, and Mom Margie not only for coming to support me, but for renting a home so my family could enjoy our privacy. Thanks especially to Dad and Jude for staying so long and organizing meals for me, and to Margie for taking care of David when he needed her most.

Thanks to my dearest friend, Barbara, who nurtured me perfectly with her calm, sweet soul, even helping me step into my first postsurgery shower (the most frightening and enjoyable one of my life); thanks to my best pal, "Queen Al," who helped create the vital garden that gave me so much more to live for, and who, with Margie, made my homecoming seem like crawling into a *lavande* womb; so much love to Lorrie, who flew across the nation to nurse me with passion and magic meringue mushroom cookies; appreciation to my beloved cousin, Barbara, who connected me with vital resources and cooked up a *geshmak* chicken barley soup that Nana would have been proud of; to Nasús, for music that sang the language of strength and hope; to Roxanne, whose pajamas bathed me in soft love and whose gift of *How to Heal* soothed David's soul; to Jo Ellen, whose friendship and introduction to David Jablons brought much comfort; to Alan Newman for his encouragement and advice; to Heidi and Cindy, whose presents started arriving almost immediately; to Give Something Back Business Products, especially Alma, for gift boxes brimming with life; to Dale, whose organization, The Cancer League, named a grant in my honor; to the KTOP crew, Kymberli and Eco-Kind, who gifted me with professional housecleanings; to Roseanne and Lizzie for the beautiful love letters and prayers that strengthened me; thanks to the Calthorpes and Calthorpe Associates, whose solicitude and generosity assuaged so much fear; and to all my other friends, family, neighbors, religious community (especially Harry, Pamela, and Carol), and clients who sent cards, flowers, gifts, meals, prayers, and, most important, love.

And, of course, all my gratitude to Dr. Aye, Jill, Dr. Mountain, Dr. Granelli, Maria, and my other health care providers whose astuteness and great skill helped keep my spirit and body alive so I could write this book.

Finally, thanks to Missy for teaching me so much about friendship before she died, and all my love to Billee for the bittersweet blessing that helped give me one of the two people I live for most.

—July 22, 2003

Thank you for helping me write

Without Kirsty Melville at Ten Speed Press, *Help Me Live* would not be. She planted the seed, and I was blessed to be the one to water it. Kirsty, I cannot thank you enough. And as for current publisher, Lorena Jones, I cannot think of anyone brighter and more perfect to harvest the seed. Thanks especially to my editor, Meghan Keeffe, whose critical eye kept my heart in the right place, whose sharp mind kept me in focus, and whose gentle prodding moved me forward. I am deeply grateful to Nancy Austin, whose design and cover photograph reveal not only great talent, but also great compassion.

Thank you to Hope Edelman, Elizabeth Kaplan, and Susan Chernak McElroy for their encouragement and counsel; to Kathy Westin, who shepherded me through writer's block and calmed my chaos; to my dear friend, Ellice, who walked with me weekly through my fears and who, by giving me permission to stop, enabled me to finish; and to my support group, especially Irene and Vicky, who bolstered me with compassion, love, and laughter.

This book would not have been possible without those who helped me find cancer patients and survivors to interview. Thanks especially to Eve Harris, Mimi Roth, and the Ida and Joseph Friend Cancer Center; the Women's Cancer Resource Center; The Wellness Community; The Cancer League; and The Breast Cancer Fund. Thanks to those who helped distribute my Survey Monkey survey (www.surveymonkey.com) and who took the survey, sometimes braving painful memories to do so.

My gratitude flows to Shelly, for opening me up with Julie Cameron's *The Writer's Way* and the concept of personal writing retreats, and to Anna, whose unwavering support enabled me to shift my spotlight of concentration back and forth between *Bay Area Business Woman* and *Help Me Live*.

Thanks to LaBertha Blair and Rabbi Jerome Grollman for encouraging me to write; to Mom, for showing me the fun and levity of language; and to John, whose talent inspired me.

I want to also thank the experts who shared their expertise and experiences with me, especially Halina Irving, Dr. Jeff Kane, and Dr. Lawrence LeShan.

Thanks to *The Sun* for its "Sunbeams" on writing; I read them before each writing session and they reassured me every time, and thanks to the retreat centers—New Camaldoli, the Mary and Joseph Center, the Quaker Center, Santa Sabina, the St. Placid Priory Center and Villa Maria del Mar—and Amtrak's Coast Starlight, which provided the peace, safety, and quiet to allow so much pain and joy to flow through me.

Most important, my deepest gratitude to all of you who shared your stories—stories that, hopefully, will help many others live longer and richer lives.

⊒⊒⊒

Finally, I must offer some apologies, as well as thanks. Although I have changed most of the details of the stories and many of the names, you may see yourself in this book. If I discuss my own or someone else's smarting because of your words or actions, please know all is forgiven. I only ask that you forgive me, as well. This book is not meant to hurt. It is meant to help. It is written with love.

Once more, I offer my most profound gratitude to all of you who have helped me to live and to write this book.

Each one of you is a miracle.

preface

> The bitterest tears shed over graves
> are for words left unsaid and deeds left undone.
>
> —Harriet Beecher Stowe

I THOUGHT I UNDERSTOOD CANCER. As a medical reporter, documentary producer, and caregiver, I had seen it from myriad sides.

Having interviewed dozens of doctors and scientists, and having read scores of articles about the scourge that will strike one in three women and half of all men during their lifetime, I thought I knew plenty.

In the process of making two documentaries about right to die issues, I had metaphorically stepped into the shoes of men and women whose lives and deaths I had chronicled. I had gazed into eyes, young and old—some fearful, some peaceful, some tear-filled—and listened to strikingly different stories of diagnosis, hope, and recovery.

I remember the gray skin of my cousin Barbara's face as she emerged from her breast biopsy and told me she had cancer. Sucked into the hurricane of medical appointments during the next few weeks, I came to understand the importance of knowing how to ask questions of busy and sometimes distracted doctors.

When one of my most beloved friends, Missy, was diagnosed with colon cancer at forty-three, I honed my research skills in the halls of San Francisco's finest medical libraries. Like a ferret, I rooted out information about treatments and clinical trials, even crossing the Mexican border and entering colorful, humid, and eerily quiet shiny-floored adobe clinics to investigate alternative therapies.

When another cousin, my best childhood friend Billee, underwent a bone marrow transplant to rid her body of breast cancer, the sterile smell of a darkened hospital room stayed embedded in my nose. I internalized the fear of death that only cancer can instill.

Indeed, I believed I knew cancer.

But in 2002, when I was diagnosed with cancer myself at the age of forty-eight, everything I thought I understood flew out the window. The magic carpet I did not even know I had been riding throughout my privileged life abruptly stopped, and I found myself in a free fall, not knowing when, where, how, or even whether I would land.

That proverbial "fall from innocence"—the innocence of believing I would live forever—began during a routine checkup, when my doctor felt a mass in my abdomen.

"It's probably nothing," Dr. Aye said, "but with your history, we should check it out."

I had uterine fibroid tumors, and I was terrified that they had grown too large to be contained and would have to be removed surgically.

That ended up being the least of my worries. Though a CT scan revealed that my abdomen was clear—oh, how my husband and I celebrated after the halo-headed radiologist held my hand and told me I was only constipated!—I received a phone call from Dr. Aye a couple of hours later.

"The radiologist took a second look, and saw something on your lung."

A biopsy confirmed what I already knew in my heart: I had lung cancer.

Even though over the past two decades I had heard countless inspiring tales of survival and had seen firsthand dozens of success stories, and even though I knew diagnosis did not equal death, I still feared that that would be my fate.

And many people treated me that way. Though I knew my friends and family wanted to help—and most did, with words and acts of great and deep compassion—some unwittingly said and did things that did not make me feel better. Words meant to assuage my fears sometimes exacerbated them. Stories intended to raise my spirits sometimes lowered them. Suggestions meant to smooth my road sometimes added bumps, dug potholes.

"Did you smoke?" [Yes, but I quit almost twenty years before my diagnosis.]

"My aunt Becky died of lung cancer, but she was much older than you."

"Are you afraid you'll die and leave your son without a mother?"

And it wasn't just friends and colleagues who seemed to develop "foot in mouth" disease. Doctors contracted it, too.

"Although your tumor is very small, and we can't see any others on the CT scan, they could open you up on the operating table and find lots of tiny tumors too small to be detected by the scan."

When I heard those words, fear, doubt, and anxiety shot through my psyche like poison. I could only hope the cancer had not spread like that through my body!

222

I realized that although I knew a lot about the disease itself, I did not know as much about people and communication as I thought. Talking with others in my post-cancer treatment support group months after my surgery (which was successful—there were no signs the cancer had spread), it became clear that my experiences were far too common. Though we laughed about the sometimes hilarious faux pas that friends, colleagues, relatives, and even strangers had committed (after all, who *hasn't* blurted out something they wish they could take back?), our pain was deep, and we felt sad that we were often too shy, frightened, or considerate to share information about words and deeds that would really help.

That's why I decided to write this book. While it may be impossible to empathize if you have not had cancer yourself, it *is* possible to sympathize and have compassion. But even that is not enough. We all need information to ensure we communicate effectively—not to say the "right thing," but to get the desired result: to make those who are ill feel better rather than worse.

I started interviewing others who had had cancer. I found counselors and therapists who had listened to hundreds of cancer patients' stories. I sought out the nation's most revered experts—people whose life work has involved studying psychology, social work, conventional and mind-body medicine, and the power and nuance of words—and I surveyed and interviewed scores of cancer patients and survivors.

With a great deal of assistance, I wrote *Help Me Live: 20 Things People with Cancer Want You to Know.*

The purpose is not to show what's right and wrong, because we are in fact all different and what is a salve to one is a scrape or stab to another. (If the objective had been to direct people, I would have called the book,

"Twenty Things to Say or Not Say to People With Cancer.") Rather, the book is designed as food for thought: Here stories unfold, providing examples of words and deeds that have helped and also those that have harmed people with cancer.

Although everyone experiences the disease differently, most share many of the same feelings. We go through similar stages, albeit in different order and for different durations: denial, anger, bargaining, depression, and acceptance. Most feel afraid. Most don't want pity, with its implied superiority. Most want to maintain control in the midst of the out-of-control growth of cells that often can be neither seen nor felt.

You may know much of the material in this book, but I hope reading it provides some reassurance. Perhaps you will read it before someone you love is diagnosed, or perhaps you will read it when someone you love is diagnosed with another serious illness or is suffering emotionally or physically.

How I wish I had read a book like this when my cousins, Barbara and Billee, and my friend Missy had cancer. How I wish I had understood the power my words wielded when I interviewed terminally ill patients intent on ending their own lives. And how I wish I had better known how to provide comfort when my mother was dying.

Hopefully it is not too late to help others in their stead, others who suffer not only from cancer, but from any disease—physical, mental, or spiritual.

Many people, myself included, are able to find the gifts of such diseases. (But please *do not ever* tell a cancer patient that his or her disease is a blessing; see chapter 16.) It may sound clichéd, but because it has helped make every moment more dear, every taste and texture more delicious, every fragrance more intense and lasting, cancer has been a gift to me.

I would also like my cancer to be a gift to you. The goal of this book and of all those who have contributed to it is to make the most uncomfortable of situations if not comfortable, then at least bearable. It asks the questions most of us are too polite or afraid to ask. Hopefully, it will help you communicate more clearly, respectfully, and lovingly. And that may help your loved one in more ways than expected.

Numerous studies have shown that cancer patients who receive emotional support live, if not longer, then at least happier lives. A pivotal 1989 study by Stanford University psychiatrist David Spiegel showed that women with metastatic breast cancer who attended a support group lived almost twice as long as those without such support. Another study—led by UCLA professor Fawzy I. Fawzy, MD—showed that melanoma survivors who participated in a six-week structured psychiatric group intervention lived longer. Though another recent study published in the *New England Journal of Medicine* showed that participation in a support group did not improve survival among breast cancer patients, study participants did report feeling better emotionally and said they felt less physical pain.

A big part of providing support involves allowing people who are suffering to express themselves. As Dr. Spiegel said of physicians, "We're trained to treat crying as bleeding, to apply direct pressure to stop it." But he says that in the case of emotions, that may not be appropriate. When training support group leaders, Spiegel says, "If you see somebody crying, don't just do something—stand there."

By standing there, you may, indeed, help your friend, wife, partner, husband, coworker, sibling, or other family member live. Thank you for caring enough to read this book. My hope is that it helps you find the words—and the silence—to show how deeply you care.

introduction

It's all very simple, or else it's all very complex,
or perhaps it's neither, or both.

—Ashleigh Brilliant

I AWAKEN IN MY DORMITORY-SIZE room at the St. Placid Retreat Center and can hardly wait to peek outside at the thin-limbed maple tree, its wide five-fingered leaves waving slowly up and down as if fanning royalty. The 6 A.M. green grays will soon glow with reflected light from the sky, and coffee calls.

What a thrill to be on my own with absolutely nothing to do but finish the final chapter of this book!

On a private writing retreat at a wooded monastery in Lacey, Washington, I am high on life, as they used to say in the '60s. Having survived cancer, I have just returned from "Cancer as a Turning Point," a free conference that freshened my heart with hope. My nineteen-year-old son, Brett, has recently called on my cell phone to ask if I know anyone who would like a newspaper subscription, which he wants to purchase out of compassion for the lackey outside Safeway who is selling them. And my husband, David, has left a voice mail, saying with love rich as mocha fudge, "I miss you so much." It doesn't get much better than this.

As I move through the dappled teal-and-purple-carpeted hallway in my slippers, I step gingerly to avoid disturbing the other retreatants sleeping behind doors labeled for Benedictines such as Heloise, Leoba, Mechtild, and Hrotsvit of Gandersheim.

In the modern fluorescent-lit communal kitchen that still smells of microwaved popcorn from the night before, I quietly turn a jar-size stainless steel knob next to the faucet. After pumping hot water into the plastic filter to brew my espresso-roasted go-juice, I leave the kitchen, silently shutting the door behind me, and tiptoe back down the hall.

Laptop cradled tightly against my left ribs—ribs that were split apart two years ago so a lobe of my lung could be removed—I enter the propped-open door labeled "Parlor" across the hall from the room named for Hadewijch (who, by the way, penned the words, Love conquers all things). I set my computer on the red-checked gingham loveseat and bend to lift the brass doorstop.

I close the door so I can tap-tap-tap on my keyboard without disturbing the man in Hadewijch, who is just eight feet away. I have met him and his egg-shape body. His black suspenders hold up gray pants, and a quarter-inch elastic strap attached to his tortoise-shell spectacles reaches around his bald head, securing his glasses to his face. With his silver beard and eyebrows and plaid flannel shirt, he looks like a cross between a leprechaun and a lumberjack. He recently lost his wife of fifty years; walking with his head down last night, he appeared to badly need some rest.

Safe in the well-insulated parlor, my fingers type automatically and with impunity to the background of my laptop's electronic whir. Deep in thought, calm and focused, a loud *KAPLUNK!* instantly raises my pulse from 60 to 120.

The door, which I had closed so gently that it had not even made a click, had not closed completely. Gravity or some other natural law had asserted its rule to complete the action.

If it had been able to talk, this is what the heavy hunk of wood might have said to me: "The road to hell is paved with good intentions! Due to circumstances beyond your control—nature, nurture, whatever—you have and may continue to unintentionally disturb people you wanted to avoid hurting at all cost!"

I relax into a quiet laugh and ask myself, "Okay, so what then is the point of having written a book about how to avoid exacerbating the pain of people who have cancer? Since you will likely hurt them anyway—since they may hear words differently than you intended them or may attach a different meaning to your actions—why even try?"

What's the point?

In deciding how to act or in choosing what to say or not to say to people with cancer, we rely on advice or examples presented by role models from childhood on. We emulate them. Real-life people and events, fairy tales and stories, movies, television, newspapers, and even comic books model what works and what fails; all inform us and show us how to act, teaching us right from wrong.

The problem is, we do not live in a world of immutable right and wrong, black and white; rather, we make our way through a spectral universe that is much broader, richer, and more brilliant than most of us have the imagination or patience to visualize.

So, if there is no ultimate right or wrong in the realm of behavior, why write a book about what to say, do, not say, and not do to make people with cancer feel better? Obviously, what comforts one may crush another. Age, diagnosis, prognosis, gender, and cultural background determine each of our unique reactions. And everyone has a different psychological makeup. As eighty-four-year-old author and researcher Lawrence LeShan, PhD, known as the "father of mind-body medicine," says, "Any therapist who treats everyone the same is a narrow, bigoted robot!"

In addition, people differ not only from each other but within themselves, depending on the time of day, month, or season—including the date of their next doctor's appointment or any number of anniversaries or special occasions. Plus, people do change. (I disliked being called *cute* when I was a teen, but as a middle-aged woman, I now delight in such a youthful description.)

In the case of cancer, especially, patients change drastically during the different phases of diagnosis, treatment, and posttreatment. Cancer itself often causes little if any pain, at least during the early stages. But treatment can make people dog sick and bone tired; chemotherapy makes some patients feel like they have downed bad sushi or been KO-ed by a brutal flu. After completing treatment, many people report feeling heady with freedom and gratitude one day but unable to climb out from between the safety of their sheets the next.

Because so many variables present themselves, the purpose of this book, is not to prescribe specific words or behaviors but to open a world of possibilities, to give you pause for thought, to share stories that will at times inspire you or make you chuckle or scratch your head.

The main objective of this book is to help people with cancer feel and heal better. But another goal is to make you, the "walking well," feel better, too. Virtually everyone shares the goal of wanting to help those in need, and we all want to feel we're doing the right thing. Very few of us would ever intentionally hurt anyone for any reason other than self-defense. And we would positively shrink in disgust from the idea of kicking someone when he or she is down.

Yet we sometimes stuff our feet in our mouths, often without even knowing it. I know I do. It usually happens when I'm in a hurry—a hurry to help, to respond, to express myself, to feel validated or comfortable. It happens when I am scared. Or happy. It happens when I, for whatever reason, neglect to think before acting or speaking, or when I cannot seem to control an impulse to blurt.

Why don't people with cancer just tell us what helps and what hurts?

If people with cancer do not want to hear why they should think positively or how awful chemotherapy is, why don't they just assert themselves and ask us not to say such things? If they don't want advice, why don't they just say so? Many people, whether they have cancer or not, fear hurting others.

"You may believe that saying no means you never get another chance with that person," writes psychologist Suzanne C. Saul, PhD, in her article, "Just Say No—Why Is That So Difficult?" She continues, "You may believe that saying no is not OK because it is rude. You will hurt the other person's feelings and that will make you bad. Both of these beliefs can be self-fulfilling prophesies. However, both beliefs are erroneous."

Therapist Halina Irving says cancer patients are not only afraid of hurting others, they also lack emotional strength because they are traumatized.

"All this talk today about patients needing to be proactive, well that's well and good, but to ask someone to be proactive at a time they are least able to be aggressive and assertive is very, very difficult because we regress more to a state of dependency."

Why not just follow the golden rule?

I am a jigaholic. Put me in front of a jigsaw puzzle and you might need a tow truck to drag me away.

On one of my writing retreats, I found a puzzle of Norman Rockwell's famed painting, "Do Unto others as You Would Have Them Do Unto You," which appeared on a 1961 *Saturday Evening Post* cover. It shows people of a range of ethnicities, ages, and religions standing together; some are pressing their palms in prayer (mainly the children); some hold native tools or sacred objects such as beads; some look up, some look down, but only two look directly at the viewer: a young black girl and her father.

Once I began assembling the pieces, I did not stop. I needed to make it all fit together, to make order out of chaos, meaning out of bits and pieces of seemingly meaningless images.

I knew there were pieces missing, because someone had scrawled that warning in blue ballpoint ink on the puzzle box. I considered giving up several times, because, after all, who wants to put together a jigsaw puzzle with missing pieces? But I could not—or would not—stop.

All along, I admired the beautiful faces—the brown, tan, pink, and yellow complexions; the eyes and noses of varied shapes; the full and thin pale and red-orange lips; the smooth, freckled, and leathered skin—and I contemplated the Golden Rule.

At the end, it all fit together.

I awoke the next morning and picked up the puzzle box. For some reason, I turned it over, and discovered a several-paragraph explanation of the Rockwell illustration: "The Buddhists say, 'Hurt not others with that which pains yourself.' The apostle Matthew wrote, 'Whatsoever ye would that men should do to you, do ye even so to them.' In the Jewish Talmud we find, 'What is hurtful to yourself, do not to your fellow man.' And in the Hindu Mahabharata, 'Do naught to others which if done to thee would cause thee pain.'"

"It's so simple," I said to therapist Halina Irving, who not only survived the Nazi Holocaust but also the attempted annihilation of her body by a particularly lethal form of cancer. "Why don't people just follow the Golden Rule? Then they'd never hurt people who've had cancer?"

"We don't always know what we would want under those circumstances," she responded, not missing a beat. "I've had a number of people say to me, 'If I get cancer I won't get treatment, I'll just call it a day.' Well, when they get cancer, they don't call it a day. I think this is the one experience you have to have lived to really know what you would do."

Or what you would want.

That's why I have chosen a chorus of diverse voices—some you will relate to, some not—to sing you a symphony of sometimes cacophonous stories. Hopefully they will resonate with you and maybe even make you want to dance.

What you will find along the way

What follows are tales, simple tips and practical suggestions based on my experience and those of scores of other people. Surveys and interviews with patients, caregivers, psychotherapists, counselors, social workers, researchers, and doctors provide sundry perspectives and sometimes contradictory information. For instance, most cancer patients and survivors say they would rather be the one to bring up the subject of their health, but some feel insulted when their friends ignore it—like an elephant in a room that no one wants to talk about. (If you pay close attention, you can usually discern what your friend wants. Or you can ask, "Would you rather I not bring up your illness?" See chapter 6.)

In addition to stories of situations told in narrative form, you will read in the margins statements from cancer patients and survivors collected through the Internet and other surveys. Throughout the book, you will hear from people newly diagnosed with cancer; people young, old, and in-between share words that have helped them; men and women with different kinds of cancer tell their stories; therapists of diverse backgrounds and disciplines offer suggestions about how to best express concern and love during a time that is often awkward for everyone.

One of the first experts you will meet works in the field of communications. After all, if this is to be a book about communicating with people with cancer, who better to call upon than those who understand the subtle nuances of words and intonation?

Learning how to follow

"The big message is that the healthy person interacting with the sick person must learn how to take communicative lead," said Lisa Sparks, whose fifty-eight-year-old father died of lung cancer when she was a graduate student.

Now with a masters degree and PhD in communications, Sparks teaches at George Mason University, writing and lecturing about how to take cues from others and react accordingly, and is also the director of graduate studies and editor of *Communication Research Reports*.

I asked Dr. Sparks what "taking the communicative lead" means.

"You listen. You shut up and listen!" she exclaimed.

That often means waiting for the cancer patient or survivor to bring up the subject rather than introducing it yourself. Once the conversation about cancer has begun, however, Sparks said we can practice communication techniques shown to smooth rather than ruffle feathers. Saying things like "It's not fair" makes the patient feel less responsible for his or her illness (and as you'll find later, many cancer patients have a secret theory about why they got cancer, which often involves being personally culpable).

"That's what we call *equivocal communication,* sort of a neutralizing message. That's a good strategy. It doesn't always work, but it's a good starting point."

Sparks said the most important principle of communication is audience analysis. Who are you dealing with? She gave an example.

"One of my colleagues has cancer right now," she began. "He was diagnosed with colorectal cancer six months ago, and it's third stage, which means it's metastasized somewhere locally and will show up again. And he's a major smoker. And he's not going to quit." Remembering that Dr. Sparks's father died of lung cancer, and that I could too, my heart ached.

"So, of course, I know all the literature," she continued. "I could be a know-it-all, of course, but I'm not. And I just have to remember my audience."

A private person, Sparks's colleague does not want to talk about his cancer, but loves talking about his teaching and the goings-on within his department. He also loves junk food and drinking.

"So I leave all these funny messages on his machine, just randomly, I'll say, 'Hey I'm at Burger King. If you're having a bad day and don't feel like cooking, this place is fantastic!' And I leave these messages just trying to make him laugh. And then I gave him a bottle of port, because I know he likes it and he survived his chemotherapy round. Anyone who can survive that deserves to celebrate."

Finally, Sparks added, "And when I talk to him, I don't ever bring up the cancer. And if he brings it up, I listen. I shut up and listen."

Sparks thinks it's easier for her colleague to spend time with her than others because she does not judge or attempt to control him.

"You'd think I'd be saying, 'Read this, read that, here's this article,' but I don't do any of that. Because of that, I think he respects me even more as a human being, knowing that I'm just a friend. I'm not buying cigarettes for him, but he still smokes and he's always going to. I'm not telling him, 'Don't smoke.'"

By watching and listening to her colleague, Dr. Sparks has learned what he wants and needs. And that's what this book is all about. Though the stories differ significantly, virtually all the characters want the same things: to be cared for and to feel understood and respected.

It's not just what you say *or* how you say it

Actions can indeed speak louder than words. Up to three-quarters of human communication takes place nonverbally according to *The Caregivers Handbook* by Jim and Joan Boulden, and you can learn to better read face and body language.

Psychology professor and renowned nonverbal communication expert Paul Ekman wrote the book, so to speak, on facial expressions. He's actually written thirteen books, one of them the classic, *Telling Lies,* which studies the hundreds of facial muscles and expressions that reveal whether we are telling the truth or not

In his most recent book, *Emotions Revealed: Recognizing Faces and Feelings to Improve Communication and Emotional Life,* Ekman delves into emotions such as sadness, anger, surprise, fear, disgust, contempt, and joy. Certain feelings are very difficult to hide, such as sadness. Sadness is particularly hard to hide—or fake—because when someone is sad, his or her eyebrows angle up in a way that few can imitate deliberately.

However, you can learn to recognize genuine emotions, and even microexpressions, which Ekman defines as "very fast facial movements lasting less than one-fifth of a second [and] and are an important source of leakage, revealing an emotion a person is trying to conceal."

"If you read it in their face," Ekman said, "then you should resonate with the emotion they're feeling to show you not only recognize it but you feel it to some extent."

Ekman said resonating, or reverberating—in other words, feeling some of what the other person feels and restating it—can be extremely difficult. "People having any severe problem, going through a divorce, for instance—what do you say to them? Should you say, 'Better it's happening now than ten years from now'? That's not what you should say; you want to have the emotional empathy to reverberate what they're feeling and allow them to talk about the feelings."

Although it can be helpful to be able to read someone's face and know what they are feeling and reverberate that, it isn't always that simple.

"Emotions never tell you their *cause,*" explained Ekman. "When you see anger in a patient, you don't know if it's anger about being sick or the fact that her friends are abandoning her or the fact that the nurse didn't show up for thirty minutes. You have to find that out, and say, 'You're upset; it looks like something's driving you nuts, and we need to talk about it.'"

But it's not always safe to be so direct.

"When I saw a microexpression on a friend's face when I was visiting him after he had open heart surgery," Ekman said, "the most I would say is 'Everything okay? Anything you want to talk about?' because if it is a microexpression, they're either unaware of how they're feeling or they're very much aware of it, but they're trying to conceal it."

Relying on the words of others

In spite of the importance of body and facial language, this book depends primarily on written and spoken language to communicate which words and actions have helped and hurt cancer patients and survivors.

In interviewing and surveying individuals, I asked if there were certain things they wanted people to know about them. Once you know what those things are, you may find it easier to think before speaking—or you may learn to say nothing at all, except with your arms, open to embrace a shocked or weakened body, or your eyes, open to acknowledge and accept someone's anguish.

Throughout this book you will be a fly on the wall in the lives of people who share a class of disease, but who sport their own idiosyncrasies. Even though there are hundreds of different kinds of cancer and each is unique, certain cancers and circumstances have their own hot buttons, and you will find them explained in the appendix. Cultural factors may also come into play, though it can be dangerous and difficult to generalize. (You might find that among older Chinese individuals, for example, a cancer diagnosis carries a stigma. Some Chinese consider the disease contagious and, therefore, may avoid cancer patients. We do that to a certain extent in mainstream American culture, too, though more subtly. One African American I interviewed claimed that hair is more important to black people than to others, so chemotherapy can be particularly devastating. But who is to say a blonde woman will mourn any less when her straight hair falls out in clumps?)

This book is not meant to be prescriptive, but descriptive. It's not here to tell you *what* to do or say; it's here to describe what others have said that helped or hurt *them.* The people who were interviewed, like the role models of your childhood, paint a rainbow of possibilities.

Help Me Live is meant to make you think; to realize that what comes out of your mouth is born in your brain and your heart and your history, and you can keep it there if you want. Do you ask someone with lung cancer whether they smoke, because you used to smoke and fear you too could get cancer? Do you ask a vegetarian how they could have gotten colon cancer after having eaten all those vegetables and legumes, feeling secretly relieved because you regularly eat red meat? Do you tell a cancer patient that you know someone else with cancer who just died, because you don't know what else to say and feel uncomfortable simply putting a hand on top of theirs and saying something plain but comforting like "It's not fair" or "I'm so sorry" or "There, there"?

The stories you will read will show you that, when someone has cancer, what is most important is to think about *them,* not about how you relate to them or to their disease. It is not about saying something wise or intelligent or compassionate. It is about saying what the patient needs to hear. He or she is facing the battle of a lifetime, and your support is needed, maybe desperately.

In talking with hundreds of patients, survivors, doctors, and caregivers and in conducting an Internet survey, I collected myriad phrases and words that have made cancer patients and survivors cringe, wince, or squirm—or alternately, melt, glow, or laugh. I learned that though there is no right or wrong, there is almost always good intention. If you give yourself time to think and feel, you will do the right thing.

When I asked people with cancer what they wanted people who haven't been diagnosed with cancer to know, they came up with dozens of suggestions. Though I have condensed them to just twenty (and another twenty or so in the appendix), they are as varied as the individuals themselves. Only guidelines, these suggestions spring from the same needs. Although it's not one of the chapters in this book, "I need to know I am loved" is perhaps what people with cancer—what all people, in fact—want you to know first and foremost.

Watch. Listen. Think. Think nurture. Think comfort. Think them. Think love.

Caring for your loved one's feelings—taking in his or her pain—will not damage you. Putting yourself in someone else's shoes will remind you of how profound their situation is, perhaps lessening the import of your own problems for a while. The experience will hopefully leave you enriched for having truly given of yourself—for having helped someone live.

20 things
people with cancer
want you to know

1.

"It's okay to say or
do the 'wrong' thing."

**I have brutalized more patients by responding
lovingly and caringly in the wrong way.**

—Lawrence LeShan, PhD

LAST SUMMER, MY FRIEND ALICE was about to undergo surgery. She asked me to take her into the hospital the morning of the procedure and, after an overnight stay, bring her back home. She didn't need to ask. Al was one of my pals who was there for me all the way during my illness; she helped create the luscious garden of lavender, rosemary, chocolate mint, poppies, and thyme that makes my eyes glitter and mouth water each time I meander through my front yard; she brought me little gifts like bath gel that encouraged me to drown my sorrows in my tub; she took me for a massage soon after my body had healed from surgery but my spirit still ached with dank dreams and memories.

Alice explained why she wanted me, of all her girlfriends, to accompany her on the morning of her surgery. "I know that you can keep quiet, that you won't be yakkin' all the time!"

I awakened that morning terrified. The thought of losing her was excruciating, but I could not get the thought out of my mind. My cancer surgery (almost exactly one year before) had frightened me to my very core, even though I had undergone several other procedures dating back to an appendectomy at age fifteen. But I knew better than to share my trepidation with Alice; her surgery was a done deal.

I jumped out of bed at 5 A.M., after a night of broken sleep, and downed two cups of extra strong coffee to face the long day. Her surgery was to last into late afternoon.

By the time I reached her home at 7 A.M., I was buzzing.

"Hey! How you doing?" I asked, smiling, eyebrows raised too high.

"I'm okay." Always the polite hostess, Al proffered a cup of coffee.

"I appreciated honesty and people who said they were afraid of saying the wrong thing. Even when they did, I knew how much they cared."

—L.C., kidney cancer survivor

I should have known better, but more coffee sounded good. My hands needed something to do, and I thought gripping a cup would help me get a handle on my fear. But the third cup was too much. My nerves felt raw, and they moved my mouth incessantly.

"I'm so glad I get to be with you this morning," I chirped. "So, how you feeling? Did you see that story on the news last night about the new museum?"

Like a dog wanting to be let out to pee, I followed Alice from her kitchen to her dining room to her living room. I continued with my questions.

"What time do we need to get out of here?" "How long will it take to get to the hospital?" "Should I park in the garage or is there street parking?"

"Shhhhhhhhhhhhhhhh," Alice breathed out slowly, palms down, pushing the air in front of her face to the floor. "I need calm. I need quiet," she whispered.

I couldn't believe what I had done, knowing what a person going into surgery needs! And Alice had even said what she needed—for me to stay quiet!

Nobody's perfect

As Confucius said, "Be not ashamed of mistakes and thus make them crimes."

Dr. Jimmie Holland, a psychiatrist and former director of psychiatry at Memorial Sloan-Kettering, founded the field of psychooncology more than three decades ago. She said of mistakes (and she has heard of plenty), "I do think you can say the wrong thing and apologize and it's okay. If you say the wrong thing and realize it and say it with sincerity—'I'm really sorry, I realize that wasn't a good thing to say'—people will forgive you. They'll understand."

One cancer survivor who later became a social worker realized that her expectations of her loved ones had been too high. "Somehow I thought they should know what to do or say, and they didn't always, even though they cared and tried. Maybe what made a difference in my reactions to people was my perception that they were honestly trying to understand how I might feel."

Even if people feel hurt, most realize their friends and loved ones have good intentions. One man with cancer who answered my survey said that although he had "of course" been hurt by things people had said, he usually noticed and appreciated their efforts more than their words.

Even if the person with cancer does not fully forgive you, it is important to forgive yourself. If you do not have the opportunity to make it up to the offended friend, colleague, or family member, you can always make it up to someone else. Next time, you can make sure you think twice before opening your mouth. But Halina Irving doesn't think you should hold your tongue unnaturally.

"Anytime you suppress what you want to say, you inhibit yourself; you put up a wall between you and the person with cancer you are talking to. And if you have to start watching your words that carefully, you'll run out of words, and its going to become very tense and stilted, and the patient will feel it and will say 'I want people to treat me like me, not just like a cancer patient.'" (See chapter 12, "I am more than my cancer.")

Stilted conversation and second-guessing

I awoke just in time that morning. During a personal writing retreat in the Santa Cruz Mountains, I had promised my dear family friend Den that I would meet him thirty minutes away at his doctor's office, even though I was approaching my book deadline. Den had recently been diagnosed with cancer and had undergone surgery; he was about to learn the results of various diagnostic tests that would tell him whether the disease had spread.

Den was petrified, as was I. Den's wife, Missy—one of my best friends—had died of colon cancer seven years earlier, and we had watched her body waste away. Her spirit, however, had seemed to grow larger and larger until she almost glowed with serenity. Still, she left us. And two children, seven and nine years old. It was devastating.

I thought I had a good grasp on what to say, do, not say, and not do to help Den through his illness. But in my heart, I knew there was much I did not know and that all I could do was try to be aware, gentle, and loving.

Most of all, I feared that at some point I would say the wrong thing. Yet a phrase or platitude most others would cringe at might be just the one to assuage his fear. I pledged to myself I would hug him and try to keep my mouth shut as much as possible.

> *"I knew from having a friend with cancer how terrifying it can be. I kept that in mind when people said inappropriate things, and forgave them of course."*
>
> —S.D., breast cancer survivor

I left the retreat center and drove through the tall dark redwood forest, its clean pine scent strong and invigorating. I was nervous about arriving on time; I had planned on leaving a half hour earlier, to make sure I arrived before Den did, but I had pushed the snooze on my alarm clock and finally sprung up forty-five minutes late, with just enough time to wash, brew coffee, and run out the door.

Since Missy had died, I had seen her family frequently, even though they lived an hour and a half away. Her children were now fourteen and sixteen, and they had grown into beautiful healthy teens: Emily has her mom's straight blonde hair, as well as her light eyes. Chris is beautiful also, and his deep wisdom makes me feel like I am talking with his mom sometimes. Both children inherited Missy's keen intelligence and wit.

Den and I had remained close, too. We had all been pals since the '80s when we lived in Portland and Missy and I worked at the same television station. The bond of friendship formed by Den's and my mutual love of Missy only strengthened once she was gone.

I felt strongly that I should accompany Den to the doctor. That's pretty much rule number one: It's good for the patient to have someone with him or her at the doctor's office who can take notes, ask questions, and help the patient synthesize the information later.

But in the days before Den's appointment, I worried a bit. "I have a deadline," I thought, self-importantly. Den had told me that his old pal Gary was going with him to the doctor's appointment also, so I let myself wonder whether I was really needed. "Since Gary's going, maybe I should wait until the next time, when I can be of more use," I rationalized. "Gee, I really want to see the kids, too, so it would be better if I just went for a visit Friday night, after my retreat."

"It wasn't so much the specifics of what people said or did, but the feeling that accompanied their words or actions."

—J.U., breast cancer survivor

What?!? My dear friend, and the husband of one of the best friends I ever had—the father of two children I love like family—was just diagnosed with cancer and he was to learn that morning whether there was any sign that it had spread.

Thanks in part to my friend Ellice, who had advised, "Of course, you should go with Den!" I shut up my inner whiner and drove off down the mountain at 7:30 A.M. ("We go kicking and screaming towards enlightenment," said Dr. Jeff Kane).

As I rounded the first sharp turn in the narrow road, I saw a blackbird the size of a football in a tree to my left. I noticed his black back shimmer in a slim ray of sunlight, and he took flight, hovering maybe fifteen feet above the asphalt that split a path through the thick redwood grove. The bird continued to coast like a seaplane with four-foot wings just yards in front of me for another half mile. It was one of the most beautiful sights I had ever witnessed.

"Thanks, Missy," I said aloud.

I arrived fifteen minutes before Den and my appointed meeting time and welcomed the luxury of being able to read a couple of booklets from the retreat center on Quakerism, about which I knew little. Soon Den and Gary arrived. When Den walked into the waiting room and saw me, I saw relief and maybe a flash of joy. We enjoyed some mighty hugs, first Den, then Gary. I hadn't seen Gary since Missy's funeral almost seven years ago to the day. It had been a day like today: clear and a perfect seventy degrees.

We made small talk, although nothing's small when you're awaiting test results. "How you doin'?" I asked Den.

"A few pins and needles here."

"Yeah, that's understandable," I said, glad I resisted the urge to say, "Don't be afraid."

While a nurse sat Den down in another room to prick his finger for a blood test, Gary and I were led to the exam room. He asked me about my own health. I started to answer, but was relieved when Den walked in so we could focus on him. His face was poppy red as he sat on the exam table, shoulders hunched and hands crossed between his knees. I felt an impulse to stand up, walk over, and put my arms around him. It felt right; I obeyed.

The doctor came in. Ready with my writing tools, I scribbled every word the doctor said as quickly as I could. I thought I had brought my micro-cassette player, but couldn't find it in my purse.

The doctor explained what he knew about the cancer and what he rec-ommended. He referred Den to a surgeon at Stanford who would explore the possibility of removing his abdominal lymph nodes to prevent the spread of the cells. The good news was there was no sign the cancer had spread already; Den's PET and CAT scans were clear, and his labs showed no evidence of hormones that indicate tumor growth.

As the doctor rattled off instructions for Den—to pick up his CAT scans from the hospital, the PET scans from another department, and the labs from yet another location—I wrote them down. Smiling reassuringly, the doctor said, "See you in four weeks. And I do believe you're going to be okay." I hoped Den had heard that loudly and clearly; I was eager to repeat it to him.

Gary and I stood up, walked over to Den, who was still seated on the waist-high exam table, and put our arms around his shoulders; we shared another bear hug. After a few seconds Gary said, "We gotta stop; I'm get-ting excited!" and we all howled with laughter. "That's why men can't hug," I said, clicking my tongue.

Gary knew instinctually what to say to Den. I loved watching their inter-action. Gary said, "What I heard the doctor say is that you're going to be okay. You're gonna be fine, pal." Den replied, "Yeah, but this really sucks." "Yeah," agreed Gary, "and I didn't really get excited."

Again, laughter. "You guys up for a cup of coffee?" I asked. "Sure!" My work could not have mattered less at that point.

I tried not to talk about my own battle with the crab, knowing that peo-ple with cancer don't want to hear about other people's experiences, but I found myself inadvertently giving advice. Having glanced at a newspaper headline about the beheading of a U.S. soldier in Iraq, I said, "When I had cancer, I stopped reading newspapers and watching the news." "You didn't want any more bad news, huh?" replied Den. And I realized, that was about me, not him.

Gary started talking about living healthfully. "Well, I guess it's a good idea to do what we should all be doing anyway—eating right, exercising . . ."

"Yeah, when I had cancer I started meditating for the first time in my life," I added, and then wondered, Are we giving advice to Den about what he should and shouldn't do? Is that what he needs?

My gut told me no, but there we were. We had already hugged. Gary told a joke. I talked a little about the challenges of parenting. I'd asked Den how work was going. Gary asked about the kids. We talked about funny movies.

When I mentioned "menopause memory" after not being able to recall the name of an actor, Gary shared that his wife was menopausal and that they were both having a difficult time coping with night sweats. I wondered whether it was upsetting for Den to hear us talk about menopause. He would have loved sharing Missy's night sweats. I would have, too.

ᗣᗣᗣ

I was so glad I went with Den that morning. Even though I may have done some "wrong" things: Did I talk about myself too much? Did I give Den too much information about a supplement I take? Why did I say how great I thought it was that he wouldn't have to go through chemo knowing that, when you're diagnosed with cancer, the only great thing is the possibility of being cured? I was there with love and good intentions.

I hoped for the courage to apologize to him for my errors in speech or judgment. I knew he would forgive me, if indeed I did say anything that made him bristle or ache.

ᗣᗣᗣ

The point is, these twenty-plus things people with cancer want you to know are meant as guidelines only. All of us say and do things that can be misconstrued or can in some way inadvertently hurt someone. That's not the problem. The problem arises when you are so afraid of making a mistake that you stay away from someone who needs you.

Make a leap of love: Listen to the person with cancer. Encourage him or her to share whatever feels comfortable. Accept your friend or loved one's feelings, even if they make you uncomfortable. And, most important, just be present.

2.

"I need to know you're here for me (and if you aren't, why not)."

It's the friends you can call at 4 A.M. that matter.

—Marlene Dietrich

THIS CHAPTER MAY BE THE MOST difficult to write, because it concerns the kernel, the seed, the center of most of our psyches and is the nexus of this book. I hope it will not be too painful to read, and I urge you to hold out for the pleasure you will hopefully come away with.

First, it is safe to say that all of us want to know that our friends and family will be there for us when we need them most, and that our deepest fear is that they will abandon us.

The truth is that people both will and will not be there when we need them most. In this chapter, the diverse tales will show how some people have been present for their friends and loved ones, and they will explain why others may have disappeared. The stories will also suggest how, if you happen to be one of those who has a difficult time dealing with people who are ill, you can still help them—or at least help mitigate the pain your conspicuous absence might cause.

⊇⊇⊇

When I called my dad and stepmother and told them I had cancer, they said they would travel from Missouri to California to stay with us for as long as

I wanted. My brother and his family wanted to drive to California from Oregon. And my husband's mother wanted to fly from Louisiana, even though her husband was very ill himself. (Luckily, I wanted to see them all, and they did ask permission before coming. But some people don't. One woman wrote to me: "My family, they live in the South, they wanted to come visit, but I just wanted peace and quiet." That's why it's important to ask permission before booking a flight. See chapter 6, "Asking my permission can spare me pain.")

In one of those amazing strokes of serendipity, there would be room enough for all our loved ones to come and stay. Our next-door neighbor, Waylon, had been renting his home from his father, Peter, since we moved in eight years ago. But Waylon had just bought his own home, vacating his father's house. Peter decided not to sell, but to keep the house as a rental investment property. It became available to rent just as I was diagnosed with cancer.

My family rented the home for one month, and it enabled everyone to come, while also affording my husband, son, and me our privacy, which we badly needed.

My best friend, Barbara, from Oregon, and my dear cousin Lorrie from Philadelphia both offered to help take care of me after my surgery so my husband could go back to work. David had missed many days in order to support me, accompanying me to every test, procedure, and doctor's appointment. I wanted him to get back to work, not only to help his employer, but so he could escape some of the stress of caregiving (see chapter 19, "I want my caregiver to take good care of herself or himself.")

The sacrifices my family and friends and neighbors were willing to make for me buoyed my spirits and made me feel deeply blessed and grateful. A couple of friends did not offer to help, but I did not even notice until I had completed treatment and fell into a fissure of depression.

In researching this book, however, I heard too many stories of men and women who felt abandoned and whose anger, sadness, and bitterness persisted for months and even years. Often the stories involved best friends and siblings; one even involved a husband who left his wife because he could not deal with her illness. His first wife had died of cancer, and he just wasn't willing or able to endure that kind of pain again.

"There are some people who can't deal with bad news; they can't deal with sick people, they can't deal with people who are losing their job, and their range is rather restrictive," psychologist Paul Ekman explained.

"When you say 'can't,' do you mean 'unable' or 'unwilling' to deal with it?" I asked, surprised. Somehow I had always thought of it as a matter of choice, but I could tell he saw it differently, and since he was a pioneer in his field, I thought it best to listen with an open mind.

"Unable to," he answered. "I think most anyone would make that choice if they could, but these people can't deal with it, they just aren't psychologically able to do it."

Ekman explained that some people don't have much of a capacity for "emotional empathy"—for feeling what another person is feeling. Others don't have much "cognitive empathy," which means intellectual understanding of how someone might be feeling. And still others have little "compassionate empathy," the desire to actually help another.

"I wanted to be with people who were present to my pain—physical and spiritual pain. Not people who had to tell me things about what they thought would make me feel better."

—T.H., Hodgkins disease survivor

Other people, of course, are pregnant with compassion. But unlike someone who is eight months pregnant with a baby, it can be difficult to recognize who possesses such empathy until you're sick and see it firsthand.

Some people I barely knew came out of the woodwork so to speak, to be there for me. It seemed surprising, but not when you consider the issue of vulnerability.

I know it was much easier for me to support my peripheral friends and relatives suffering from cancer than those closest to me, such as my cousin Billee and my dear friend Missy. It hurt more to see them hurt, and I was much more fearful of losing them. It was easier for me to be there for a neighbor that I hardly knew because, although I liked her very much, I was not struggling with my own fear of losing her, my own fear of abandonment.

But psychology aside, Ekman emphasized that the reason some people aren't there for their friends and loved ones has more to do with ignorance.

"They just don't know what to do; they don't know what they're supposed to say," he began. "Illness used to be a part of everybody's life, as part of their extended family, since they were a child—when they had aunts and uncles and grandparents around—but now, by the time friends get seriously ill, they aren't prepared, they don't know what to do."

Ekman said some people fear they will make things worse for the patient if they allow them to talk about how bad things are, when actually the reverse is true: Talking about it usually makes patients feel better. "And there are some people who think 'If we talk about it, it's just going to make it worse,' but really it just makes it worse for them, not the sick person. So you have to hope they have a lot of good fortune in their lives," Ekman laughed, "because they won't be able to deal with their own misfortunes when they occur."

His face became serious again as he continued. "We like to think that life is controllable and predictable, but the only things for sure are death and taxes . . . and with taxes, you know when it's going to occur."

Marching to mastectomy

Although Mindy Barris could not know when death would occur, she always suspected it would happen while she was still young.

"I was born here, but my dad died right after I was born, and my mother took me in a laundry basket on a train back to Ohio," Mindy explained to me over lunch at Zza's Trattoria, its red, green, yellow, and blue checkered tablecloth adding even more cheer to the sunny autumn day. "Then she died of breast cancer. So I always lived with this kind of fear in the back of my mind.

"The day I outlived my mother—my mother died when she was fifty-one—I just bought myself the best bottle of champagne in the whole world, got rip-roaring drunk by myself, and said 'Yeah! I got beyond it!'"

But eight years later, Mindy was diagnosed with breast cancer. "I had the galloping kind—the kind that was going fast," she recalled. "And they said they wanted to do a mastectomy, and I said, 'You know what? Why don't you just take them both off, and I won't have to worry about being lopsided.' My mother's cancer had traveled to the other side within a year, so why not get them both taken off at once?"

Mindy's candor and humor came as no surprise. A half hour earlier, when she had walked into my office, she had hugged me and then clutched the bottom of her tightly knit red-and-white striped sweater. She lifted it up, secured it with her chin, and pulled her bra, filled with prostheses, up over her chest.

"See? They're both gone," she exclaimed, smiling so widely that her crow's feet furrowed almost to her hairline.

"Wow," I said, disarmed. I had never before seen in the flesh a chest bare of breasts and nipples, blank like a soft shield. Though we'd met less than sixty seconds earlier, she had flashed me as if we had been pals since childhood. Perhaps I should have felt confused, but her action felt appropriate because . . . well, because of who I knew Mindy to be.

We had talked on the phone several times, and I had fallen in love with her voice, which matched her personality perfectly. Though she was sixty-eight years old, she sounded like a young Doris Day, a little raspy and very animated. When I identified myself on the phone after we had emailed a few times, she said, "Lori! Hi! Great to talk with you," and I believed her.

The first thing she told me about was her double mastectomy. "I got them both whacked off," she explained. "When I got diagnosed with cancer, I didn't go through some of the stages other women do, like the 'Why me?' stage."

"This is not some TV program. It's real. The vomit, the tiredness, the hair loss, the threat are all real. If you aren't prepared to deal with that, take a hiatus. We'll be better friends down the road than if you try to stick out what you can't tolerate just because you feel like to do otherwise means you are a bad person."

—A.S., breast cancer survivor

Face to face at the restaurant, we sat by an open window that welcomed in fresh air that was as warm as her smile, and she told me the story of her cancer diagnosis and treatment—a story that could have been terrifying, but calmed me and filled my heart with hope.

"I was absolutely terrified," she began. "But my family just pulled together. It just makes me cry to think about it."

Her thirty-five-year-old son, who lived in a nearby suburb, did all the research for her.

"I was just shell-shocked. And you don't want to appear to be self-absorbed and yakking about it all the time, and you don't know what the doctors are giving you, all this, 'Well, you could have a lumpectomy, radiation, and chemo, or you could do this or that,' but I wanted to do a mastectomy. And you don't know what to do."

Her son visited websites and emailed Mindy information, including photographs and sometimes something she needed even more—humor. "'Mom, you know, you can be any size you want to be!' he said. 'You always wanted to have big boobs. Well, now's your chance! Why don't you get ones like Dolly Parton?'"

"My husband and daughter were there for me anytime I needed them, never judging my response to things, just loving me."

—D.B., endometrial cancer survivor

Mindy's other children were there for her, too, even though they had careers and families to care for. Her thirty-three-year-old identical twin daughters flew to San Francisco from their Los Angeles homes to support her. And they helped not only her—stopping at a knitting store to buy her a hundred dollars' worth of yarn so she could keep her hands busy while sitting in doctors' waiting rooms—they also reached out to others they would never meet.

One day, one of her daughters waited with Mindy to see the doctor. "And of course she was scared the way a kid is," Mindy said, moving her face a little closer to mine, "so she tried to think up useful things to do."

Mindy's daughter noticed that there were not enough magazines in the waiting rooms. So she gathered up all her friends' spare magazines; together, Mindy and her daughter put them to good use. "We were like the magazine dolly, and we'd go around putting magazines in waiting rooms."

I remarked, "There's nothing worse than reading a *People* magazine from two years ago," but then laughed, remembering that once you have had cancer, there are many things much worse than not being able to keep up with the latest entertainment news.

Mindy laughed. "Yes, but it is especially awful when the last part of the article's been ripped out." Then she said, out of the blue, "I'm having a Tamoxifen hot flash," and explained how the anticancer drug can cause side effects.

"I'm so sorry," I said.

"Oh, don't be sorry. I'm one of the luckiest people in the world. I'm sitting here by a window, and nobody ever died of a hot flash."

But people do die in surgery, and as we spoke about the day of her mastectomy, I was flashing, too—flashing back to the day of my surgery, the most terrifying day of my life. I was glad to turn my full attention to Mindy's tale.

"They wanted me there at six in the morning," she smiled, "so I could get my weird shoes on and everything. My kids came from Los Angeles, and my son had had T-shirts made."

Emblazoned on the T-shirts was "Marching, marching to mastectomy."

"It was so wonderful; we all wore them, holding hands, walking to the hospital."

Mindy's surgery went well, but soon after, she learned the cancer had spread to her lungs, and she would need to have one of her lobes removed. Just when it seemed things could not get worse, Mindy's husband received a cancer diagnosis.

"My husband was diagnosed with prostate cancer the same day I had my lung surgery, and everyone in the family said, 'You gave it to him, Mom. That's what happens when you sleep with somebody—he gets it, too.' And then we started saying, 'Yeah, we want to go to every floor in the cancer center—breast, lungs, prostate—how many more floors are there in here?'"

Mindy was as present for her husband as he had been for her. But some people don't have loving spouses or family members as dedicated and committed as hers. And some people do not have "family" at all.

Why people disappear

"I have NO family. Dispersed and dysfunctional," Abbe wrote to me in an email. The gist of her story was about how helpful her friends had been during her two bouts of breast cancer. One girlfriend went camping with her after chemo, and, in a tender gesture, offered to rub her bald head. "It was good strokes, both physically and mentally," Abbe noted.

"The most touching thing was when I was diagnosed, one of my best friends asked, 'What time are we going to the hospital?' She stayed with me through the operation, without my asking. I had another friend who was there with me every step of the way."

But there were two people who weren't with her even an inch of the way. "I was the most hurt by my closest friend, who did the least. Ditto for my brother. He couldn't deal with the disease."

Abbe said she could understand her best friend's reaction, because the friend had lost her mother to cancer. And she realized that she couldn't change her brother. But she does believe her loved ones could have made it less devastating for her.

"What would have eased the pain of these unsupportive people would have been a verbal or written message that they're not equipped to deal with my cancer," said Abbe, trying to muster compassion herself. "Not everyone can deal with life-threatening situations, but to ignore a person without an explanation tears at the heart. This is not the time to add stress."

Andrea Adler's siblings and best friend also added stress with their unexpected absence. "My best friend, who I've had since high school, didn't call me until probably three months into my treatment, and then I had to call her," she said sadly. "Now, I knew she knew, but I think it was jut really hard for her to face. Finally I had to break that barrier.

"I had to see if this was a rejection of me or if she was just having a tough time facing it. It was more her having a tough time facing it, but in your mind you kind of think, 'Am I like a leper that people don't want to see?'"

Bay Area Tumor Institute Executive Director Barry Siegel said some people disappear because they convince themselves they don't know what to say. They tell themselves they're better off staying away so they don't cause more pain for the patients.

"We think [the patients] are already damaged goods. But all we've done for them at that point by staying away, is we've cut them off from the social interaction that makes us people."

"I loved to hear, 'I'm here whenever you need me.'"

—S.B., breast cancer survivor

Siegel, whose nonprofit agency provides information, referral, and numerous support groups, used to teach philosophy. "Aristotle said man is a social animal. Now we're going to cut him off from being a social animal because we're frightened that we're going to hurt his or her feelings, when that's really a time when greater social intercourse is needed."

Or, as author Peter McWilliams wrote in *Life 101,* "To avoid situations in which you might make mistakes may be the biggest mistake of all."

Andrea's parents came all the way from Florida for a month to help care for her and her three children. Her neighbors, employers, and friends rallied around her. Her church made sure she had meals delivered to her door every single night.

"Because I was single when this happened to me and didn't have anybody in my life, some of the most incredible gifts were massages because the only time anybody was touching me was to stick a needle in me or to examine me or give me a biopsy."

Other gifts massaged her soul. "The school gave me free tuition while I was in treatment. The lunch guy at school gave them [my children] a free hot lunch every day." When she was most ill, her children stayed with her ex-husband. "People came and drove the kids to my house after school so I could see them every day, and then their dad would pick them up at my house."

"My family (three siblings and my mother) wouldn't call or check in on me. They kept saying, 'I don't know what to do.' I would say, 'Why not ask me?'"

—C.T., breast cancer survivor

When her friends from church delivered her meals, sometimes she would find a gift card to a video store. "Just little things like that really helped," Andrea said.

How to be there without being there

There are so many ways to be there without actually being present on the phone or in person. If you have limited financial resources, you need not send a gift, just a simple letter on lined paper. Or send one of Ashleigh Brilliant's brilliant postcards (see the resources section).

The point is to let the patient know you care about them. They need to know they are surrounded by people who love them.

"Our existence is by definition a tragic one because it ends and because we know that we are finite and we will die," said therapist Halina Irving. "If someone doesn't have religious faith and believe in an afterlife, that is a very difficult condition. However, there is still one thing that makes us feel that it's worth it anyway. More than money, more than success, and more than prestige is the profound meaning and fulfillment and fullness of human relationships."

Irving said that when our lives are threatened, when we are in a state of crisis and terrible trauma, we need relationships more than ever. Though the people in our lives can cause frustration and even pain, they also enrich us.

"No matter how terrible the circumstances for a human being, to feel cared about, attended to, heard, understood, and accepted is the greatest gift we can give that human being—the only solace, the only comfort." And our reward for giving comfort and solace is personal gratification and joy.

It's never too late

Even if you have not been able to be present as much as you would have liked for a loved one with cancer—for whatever reason—you may find your situation changed after the person has recovered. It is never too late to show up. And if you are a cancer patient or survivor reading this, it is never too late to ask someone why they were not there for you in the way you wanted. Sometimes a simple misunderstanding is to blame. Or perhaps someone was following the Golden Rule, assuming that what they would want in your situation is what you wanted. Or maybe they trusted that you were close enough to ask for what you needed. That is what happened to me during the winter of 1999.

Though the San Francisco Bay Area rarely chills to freezing, I seemed to spend that late California winter trapped on an iceberg. Although we had just rejoiced in my son's Bar Mitzvah and I had begun an exciting new job, I was facing two impossible impending losses: that of my mother and that of my dog, who I credited with saving my life when I was a workaholic documentary producer.

"Neglect is just as painful as harsh, judgmental words, especially when it comes from people I have supported in tough times."

—J.B., lymphoma survivor

My mother was dying of emphysema. My brother had recently transferred her from her comfortable skylight-cheery independent living center to a nursing home, where she would receive hospice care. Just a few days after Brett's Bar Mitzvah, I flew up to Oregon to spend the last eight days of Mom's life with her, sleeping on an inch-thick foam pad atop a shiny cold tile floor. The room was lit with one small lamp; the ceiling light remained off except when the nurses squeaked in to check vital signs or give injections. Outside the window, the rain painted everything dark blue by day, black by night.

A woman with whom I had recently grown close, Terry, sent a huge rainbow assortment of flowers in a grass green vase to our nursing home room. They replaced the generic antiseptic smell with a distinctive fresh fragrance. Although my mother could not see the pink lilies and red roses, I knew the aromas nestled in her nostrils, providing solace and pleasure.

When I returned home after Mom's difficult death—her regression to childhood, her hellish nightmares, her wasting away so much that when I hugged her I felt not flesh but a sharp scapula—we learned that our beloved dog, Griffin, had an untreatable and inoperable brain tumor.

No moon illuminated the sky the night he died. No stars shone as we wept outside in the cold, placing his still sweet-smelling body in the car to be taken away.

⊒⊒⊒

After Mom and Griffin died, and after my new position pulled me farther away from my home office, where I had spent most of my time working, Terry and I grew apart. Our friendship had been deteriorating anyway; it was based mainly on our children. Even so, her sudden disappearance left me bereft. Although I stopped calling her, I needed her to continue calling me.

I was so busy with my new job, travel, consulting work, and running the household, that I didn't dote on it. But my sorrow persisted, a subterranean ache.

Though the precise reason for the death of my friendship with Terry remained a mystery, I could not let my pain remain hidden from my dearest friend, Barbara, who has been there for me since our college days when we became soul sisters.

Barbara called often during that winter to check in on me. With the soft voice and kind but firm tone of a highly skilled elementary school educator, she probed gently. Though her kindness never waned, she could not hide her disappointment when I told her I wouldn't be able to meet her for our annual winter weekend away.

For the past several years, the two of us had taken a vacation each February. But that winter, because of the Bar Mitzvah, finances, Griffin's and my mother's deaths, and my new job, I was unable to leave even for three days. I would miss that special time of renewal and intimacy, but I did not feel there was another way.

Our families did vacation together, however, the next summer in Brookings, the Banana Belt of the Oregon coast. It was the first of many shared summer retreats. We camped in a glorious area of the South Coast, within walking distance of dramatic high cliffs, clean beaches of fine sand and dark gray volcanic stone, and a healthy ocean of surf and of seals sunning themselves on rock islands offshore.

Barbara and I had slipped away from the group to share a cup of tea in a tiny pine-paneled coffee shop. It was uncharacteristically overcast outside, and I had let down my defenses for the first time in many months. My heart had healed from losing Terry, but some residual pain remained. I think I displaced what I saw as Terry's abandonment and projected it onto Barbara, wishing she had somehow been more present.

As I relaxed my body and mind from the winter's traumas, my emotions came crashing down like the waves we could hear a block away. I started crying. My tears felt like the tide, fierce and unstoppable.

"Honey, what's wrong?" asked Barbara, her dark brown eyes moistening, eyebrows arched. "Oh, sweetie, tell me."

My words rushed out chaotically. I told her it had been the worst year of my life, losing my mother, Griffin, and Terry. And I told her I had felt alone, that I had wished I could have spent time with her, that she could have comforted me more.

"I had no idea!" Barbara said, and started to cry herself. Reaching across the small dark wood table, she cupped my hand in both of hers. "I love you so much, Lori," she cried, "and I would have gotten on a plane in a second if I thought you needed me. You were so busy, and you couldn't get away for our special weekend, and you said you were doing fine."

"My best friend was there with me from the biopsy and through each and every appointment thereafter. I can't stress enough how important it is to have someone with you. Not only for support but also to think of questions you may not."

—D.D., colon cancer survivor

As her words entered my heart—as her eyes reinforced her message of love—my tears slowed to a drizzle.

"Oh, Lori. I'm so sorry. I should have asked," she continued. "I thought you would ask me to come if you needed me. I didn't want to impose. I wanted to respect your privacy. I would never, ever, do anything to hurt you!"

Barbara and I held each other, suffering and soothing, releasing and renewing. I felt horribly guilty for making her feel bad; she felt bad that I felt abandoned. We absorbed one another's tears on our T-shirts for many minutes, promising we would always ask for what we need and would not expect the other to know what that might be.

When I was diagnosed with cancer three years later, Barbara's first question to me was not, "Can I come take care of you?" but "*When* can I come take care of you?" Even though we were about to vacation together—even though Barbara was about to drive twelve hours with her family to see us, even though she hates flying—she wanted me to know she would be there, whenever I needed her, for as long as I needed her.

That helped me live. It made me want to call Terry, to find out why she hadn't remained by my side during that most difficult winter of loss. I resisted the urge, not because it was too late but because I knew it was partly my fault; I had let the friendship slip away or perhaps I had actually pushed Terry away. And I had not asked for what I needed.

The gift of an inspiring example

There is another way to be there besides actually being present. Andrea, who you met earlier in this chapter, used her aunt as an example.

"She's one of my heroes. She is a twenty-year survivor of breast cancer. And she's just the most beautiful, gracious woman, a really wonderful woman."

Not only did Andrea's aunt call and send greeting cards and letters, she gave Andrea the gift of being able to see that people do survive cancer. "When you hear the diagnosis of cancer, you think about everything you see in the movies. Everybody in the movies who gets cancer dies," Andrea observed.

But millions of people have survived cancer—nearly ten million in the United States. According to the American Cancer Society, 64 percent of cancer patients survive at least five years, and half of those with cancer live as long as those never diagnosed.

You can help people with cancer survive and live fuller lives by pointing out to them, in words and deeds, that it is possible to have cancer and go on to live a long, healthy life.

3.

"I like to hear success stories, not horror stories!"

**My words fly up, my thoughts remain below.
Words without thought never to heaven go.**

—William Shakespeare, *Hamlet*

IN THE HBO TELEVISION SERIES, *The Sopranos,* mob boss Jackie is dying of cancer. Lying in his hospital bed, weak and depressed, his pals drop in to cheer him up. Not only do they bring chocolates he literally can't stomach (he's on chemo), but one friend, Mikey, makes conversation that delivers a double punch. As he watches the nurse give Jackie an injection, Mikey warns, "Air in the line will kill 'ya!" Then he continues, "You know who else has cancer? Tony de Palma. He's got it much worse than you—it's eating his brain away!"

When Mikey leaves, Jackie shakes his head. "Thank God he left!" he sighs. "That Mikey, he's a nice guy, but he's like the Grim F-ing Reaper; it's like he knows every guy with a f-in' cancer cell, and he can't wait to tell ya!"

Nightmares can end as comedies

I have to urinate. I am looking for the restroom in a dark, crowded restaurant. I walk through a fluorescent-lit hallway and head for the door at the end. But I stop when I see the sign: Restroom for Staff Only. I walk back into the dining room, and a waiter points the way to the public ladies room. But a sign on that door reads Out of Order.

I look at the dots, lines, and numbers glowing in the darkness: 4:15 A.M. As I awaken, I try to recall details of the dream, but only the feeling of desperation remains. I get up quietly, trying not to wake my husband, David.

As I regain full consciousness, examining the dark circles under my eyes in the mirror above the bathroom sink, it all comes back to me. Not the dream, but the events of the evening; not the tastes and textures that delighted my mouth during dinner, but the taste that remains six hours later: the bitter, harsh acidity that I desperately want to neutralize.

⊇⊇⊇

Earlier that night we had gone to an Italian restaurant across the bay, becoming more relaxed as we enjoyed one delightful course after another. One of the owners came to the table to ask about our meal, and we seemed to make his day with our perfectly seasoned praise. I asked how long he had been in business.

"Twenty years," he said. And then, as if tearing open a wound, he opened his heart. He explained that his wife had died of cancer four years ago and that he still missed her daily.

"I had cancer, too," I said, wanting to soothe him. "What kind?" he asked, and when I told him, I could see from the look on his face that it was about to begin: the gushing of grief.

"That's the kind of cancer my wife had," he began. "The first time she had it, she had surgery and was fine. The tumor was contained. No chemo, nothing. But eight years later, it came back," he continued.

Having had lung cancer myself a year and a half earlier, and having had only required surgery, I pleaded in my mind, "Enough! Please, stop!" Instead, I remained silent, regarding him with deep sadness and compassion. I breathed in his pain and that of my husband, David, sitting across from me, who was perhaps feeling more terrified than I was. Eight years from now, would David be telling such a story?

"It was so horrible," the restaurateur agonized as if it had happened

"I liked hearing stories about survivors and that it wasn't a death sentence."

—B.H., lung cancer survivor

last month. "The cancer had spread everywhere; new tumors in her lung had lodged against her heart wall. She was coughing up blood; she died within a year."

The waiter arrived with a cup of minestrone, and I attempted to breathe in the soup's aroma instead of the restaurant owner's pain; I longed to taste the soup, to replace the pain with sensuous pleasure. But I could not divert my eyes from those of the widower. I was trapped in his suffering, all of our suffering, and fear flowed through me as the grief gushed from him.

"Many people want to make it seem like they can relate to what you're going through, so they tell you about people they know who have had cancer, but it does not comfort you."

—H.L., adult Hodgkins survivor

Finally he left, and David and I looked at one another, eyes round. After a moment, laughter melted the shock frozen on our faces. We smiled at the insanity of it all—of enjoying fine food in a romantic candlelit ambience while witnessing raw suffering and facing the reality that my cancer could return and claim my life as well.

We ordered a second glass of Chianti and by the time we'd finished the tiramisu, the terror of the widower's horror story was almost forgotten.

But now, six hours later, I stand wide awake in the bathroom, remembering words and images that have developed like Polaroid prints in my mind's eye: coughing up blood, gasping for breath.

The terror has returned. I scurry back to the safety of our bed. Both David and I have a long Monday ahead of us. I need more sleep to make it through the day.

I lay there for a few moments listening to my heart, wondering where— *whether*—I will be a decade from now. David awakens, as if he has heard my thoughts; he asks if I'm okay. I cry, quietly. I consider protecting him, but I so badly need comfort myself that I tell him my worries.

He holds me and whispers, "You're going to live; we're going to grow old together." I tell him how much I love him, and I get up to write so he can go back to sleep. I know I will not be able to rest until I exorcise the fear.

I huddle in the living room chair in darkness, crying softly into knees drawn close to my heaving chest. The sky lightens and the doves coo in the redwood outside the window. I relax my legs onto the floor and Franny, our heat-seeking-missile kitty, jumps into my lap. I cradle her. Our basset hound, Belle, pounds her tail against my chair, and I scratch her long soft ears.

Eight years. Is that how long I have? How to fill that time? What can be done to help me live?

And why did that man have to tell me that story, knowing I had had lung cancer and could face the same fate as his wife?

⊇⊇⊇

"His need to tell the story was greater at that moment because he's still carrying the grief," explained therapist Halina Irving, when I asked her the same thing the next day. "His need to talk about it was greater at that moment than his ability to think about you and how that would make you feel."

Irving said the reason I felt so frightened was that my diagnosis was fairly recent and it can take years to rebuild a sense of safety.

I had first heard this tall, slender woman with a slight accent (which I couldn't quite identify) on the radio. The therapist for *The Group Room*, a nationally syndicated radio show that serves as a live support group for people with cancer, struck me as not only brilliant but deeply compassionate. And, indeed, when I interviewed her for the first time that day, she assuaged my pain, partly by encouraging compassion for the man whose tale had robbed me of both sleep and hope the night before.

"We have to have a special tolerance and understanding of anyone who has suffered a loss, because the imperative to tell the story is their survival, is their healing, and that's why I believe in grief work and grief counseling. We live in a culture that doesn't allow for that."

⊇⊇⊇

Halina Irving grew up in a culture of hate and fear. Born in Poland in 1936, just before the Nazi Holocaust, she fled her homeland with her family at the age of five.

"We walked from Poland to Hungary and that's how we survived. We survived a war hiding in Hungary. Before that, in Poland, I was a hidden child, hidden by peasants while my parents were in a ghetto that had been turned into a labor camp."

Irving very clearly remembers being smuggled out of the ghetto; the difficulty of separating from her parents at such a young age haunts her still.

"One of the hardest things was that one of the peasants had a girl a little bit older than I; they took all my clothes and gave them to her, and to this day I'm a clothes horse," Irving said.

After the Russians liberated Poland and Hungary, Irving reunited with her parents and traveled to Prague. But soon they had to flee Prague as well because the Communist Party took over. From there Irving journeyed to Belgium, where she waited with her family for five years for passage to America.

That's where her training as a therapist began. Her father practiced dentistry illegally in their apartment, serving other Holocaust refugees, until they could save enough money to emigrate. Irving's bedroom served as the waiting room.

"After I was first diagnosed, we were boating with my mother-in-law and sister-in-law. They spent the entire afternoon telling me about everyone they had known who had had cancer, and telling me the details about how many of them had passed away. It made me feel terrified."

—A.L., breast cancer survivor

"I would come home from school and I would listen to his patients, who were all survivors, talk about their losses, the people they had lost," Irving said sadly. "That's how I learned about grief, because I used to sit for hours and listen to them, and I understood then about the need to repeat the same story over and over again. That's the only thing that seemed to help things: to share their stories, to talk about what they had experienced."

Once in America, Irving attended college, enrolling at the University of California at Los Angeles to study French literature. After earning her undergraduate degree, she began graduate work. It took her ten years to get her master's degree; to finance her education, she took on jobs as a teaching assistant, an associate, and a lecturer. Just before earning her PhD, she awakened from her American dream, startled.

"I found out my mother had been diagnosed with breast cancer three weeks after I took my PhD exams—they had kept it from me so I would take my exams—and for the next year and a half, I took care of her because she went into a clinical depression after her diagnosis. I took a leave of absence to go to New York, and I brought her out here to California, and my husband, John, and I took care of her."

When Irving's mother got better, she returned to New York City. "But within six weeks, she was rediagnosed with metastatic breast cancer and died," said Irving, eyes moistening. "I was spent."

"There is absolutely no way that a person who has not had cancer can fully understand the feeling of absolute vulnerability and terrorizing fear that occurs when you hear the diagnosis. It was the first time in my life that I had really thought about my own mortality."

—J.M., prostate cancer survivor

After postponing starting a family for eleven years, Halina and John Irving knew this was the time to bring new life into the world. But life would again prove ephemeral and tragic. Because of an anatomical anomaly that made it difficult for Irving to carry a child, she suffered a miscarriage during her first pregnancy. She spent her next pregnancy in bed; she carried her firstborn son to term, but he suffered from spina bifida and survived only three months.

"Loss and human suffering were part of my life from the time I was three years old," she said after relating the death of her child. I could only imagine the depth of pain she had experienced. How much more could any human being endure, I wondered.

"I had a sister who was almost ten years younger than me, and she died of a lymphoma at thirty-one," continued Irving. "First I took care of my mother, and then my baby, and then I took care of my sister when she was sick and dying.

"That experience with my sister made me feel that no matter how I was going to do it, I had to work in this field because I had experienced such pain firsthand and I had been so disappointed and truly hurt by the people whom I dealt with. As bad as the illnesses were—and the tragedies of the deaths—I wanted to be in a field where I could deal with cancer patients because I felt I had experience that would allow me not to do what had been done to us."

Irving enrolled in a master's degree program where she learned to help people deal with loss, chronic illness, disability, and death. She worked with cancer patients on the oncology floor of a hospital, offering free counseling and grief work to loved ones of people who died.

Irving's experiences as a cancer caregiver, as well as her family history of breast cancer, made her especially vigilant. When she was thirty-one, she started going in for yearly mammograms. She went to a women's breast cancer center, thinking they would be more sensitive to women who had a family history of breast cancer and would follow her closely. "And they did," Irving said, "for ten years."

But the older she got, the more scared she got so she asked for a prophylactic mastectomy. "The surgeon laughed at me and said, 'That's crazy, you don't need this. We have state-of-the-art equipment; if anything should happen we'll diagnose it so early that you'll be no worse off.'"

"I couldn't stand listening to people tell the horror stories of this aunt who died of colon cancer, or that sister-in-law's struggle with lung cancer that she lost, 'Poor dear!'"

—D.B., colon cancer survivor

Irving had annual mammograms for almost ten years, but once, eight months after her yearly visit, she felt compelled to go in for another mammogram. "For no reason—there was no lump, there may have been a little itching—I had a sense of foreboding, and I went back for another mammogram. The surgeon forgot I was coming, and they couldn't find him—this was New Year's Eve weekend—and when they found him he said, 'What are you doing here? It's too soon. After eight months nothing will show up.'" Irving almost left, but instead she insisted on another mammogram.

"And there it was," she said. The radiologist discovered Irving had lobular cancer, which constitutes only about 10 percent of breast cancers. "It's a lethal cancer, not because it's aggressive," Irving explained, "but because it doesn't form a tumor. It forms a little nucleus that you can't feel, and then it has legs that pervade the whole breast."

Lobular cancer tends to travel to the other breast, and it is very difficult to detect. So Irving requested a bilateral mastectomy. "I knew exactly what my treatment should be and they agreed, but I was very badly treated there, and I ended up leaving, having to find other doctors. That surgeon never took responsibility for the bad advice he had given me, for not informing me about the fact that there were cancers you wouldn't be able to detect early."

The happy ending to Irving's story is that she has had no sign of cancer in almost fifteen years. A successful therapist who has helped perhaps millions of ill and bereaved people through support groups and radio programs, Irving recently trained for two more years in psychoanalytic psychotherapy, and her private practice has ripened and expanded. She loves her life, and her success story serves as an inspiration to me.

⊒⊒⊒

But sitting across from Irving in an office beautifully decorated with antiques and framed heartfelt notes from patients, I still felt confused about what happened with the restaurant owner who had lost his wife. Why had I awakened in the middle of the night? Was it only that I had needed to urinate, or had the terror interrupted my peaceful sleep? And what could I do to prevent such painful incidents in the future, other than keeping my health history to myself?

Irving told me, simply and emphatically, that anyone who is not grieving, as the restaurant owner was, needs to hold his or her tongue. Conversation about losing someone to cancer is never casual.

Instead of imparting advice to me, she shared her thoughts based on decades of her own trauma, including a grim cancer diagnosis and debilitating treatment. For her, it's been a decade and a half. For me, just two years.

"The way you're existing now is the way I believe I existed, which is what we all do because we couldn't live otherwise. We go into some kind of denial—that it [dying from cancer] will not happen to us—and we push away the fact that it might happen to us, because if we thought about it we could not go on living. It would be too terrifying.

"When someone tells you about another person who has died of lung cancer—when I hear of a woman who has metastatic breast cancer after being cancer free for seventeen years—it shatters our denial, and it pulls us back, whoosh, right back to that moment of diagnosis and then treatment, when we felt most vulnerable and most in danger. After fourteen and a half years, it still happens to me, and anyone who tells you that they don't feel that is either lying or their defenses and their denial are so powerful because they're so terrified that they're not able to allow themselves to feel."

> "So many people brought out stories about people they had known with cancer. Or they brought out stories of their own aches and pains. I was not in the mood to listen to all of this."
>
> —I.S., prostate cancer survivor

At that moment, I felt an intense love for Irving. She assured me that I will survive the frightening stories I will hear, that they will even make me stronger.

Softly, she continued, "There are feelings that we cannot negate. There is no such thing as only positive feelings in your life. It is not a negative feeling to feel despair and fear under certain circumstances. Those are the natural feelings, the normal feelings with trauma, loss, loss of loved ones, and threats to our own lives."

How to treat people undergoing such trauma comes naturally if you consider what they are going through. The first emotion most cancer patients experience upon diagnosis is terror. That is partly why horror stories can devastate so quickly and why success stories of people with similar kinds of cancer can heal so tenderly.

4.
"I am terrified."

To suffering there is a limit; to fearing, none.

—Francis Bacon

HAVE YOU EVER BEEN SO frightened that you froze in your tracks? I have. I was sixteen. It was the middle of the night when my best friend, Amy, and I opened my bedroom window carefully, stepping backward out the window into the steamy St. Louis summer air. Although neither of us could see, we trusted our feet to find the top step of the ladder we had set up earlier that night.

We tiptoed through the thick Bermuda grass. Stilling our giggles with our hands, moist from excitement and humidity, we were heady with the realization that the night, just as the future, was all ours.

We ran across a blacktop road lit by fluorescent streetlights that cast huge gray orbs on the pavement, and we found our way to the Immaculata Catholic Church parking lot. Squatting in the four-foot-high space under a construction semitruck, we listened for our friends. We had planned to meet other members of "the group," as we called our clique, at 1 A.M. But instead of our friends, we met a blinding spotlight.

"Come out!" a deep voice bellowed through a speaker I could not see. To my terrified ears, the police officer sounded like God commanding me from the sanctuary just ten yards away.

I started to join my friend, who scrambled into the nearby woods, but the "Stop!" paralyzed me. Chest pounding, my terror turned to dread as the policeman ordered me into his squad car. "Where do you live?" he demanded.

"You can't take me home!" I cried, lying. "My father will beat me!"

How could I face my parents? Worse yet, how could I face the consequence of what we had done? It was early summer, and I knew I would be grounded for weeks, which, for a teen, is forever.

From that night on, whenever I imagined terror, that was the memory I summoned. The feelings, though seemingly trivial, were genuine and intense. Back then I didn't have the experience or confidence to know I could make it through that night or the summer of staying home.

By the time I was diagnosed with cancer, I had experienced many other kinds of terror: as a journalist, the fear of missing deadlines; as a girlfriend, the fear of being cheated on by one who had cheated on me before; as a lover of sweets, the fear of undergoing the pain of another root canal.

"Mostly, I wanted those close to me to just hug me and understand how frightened I was. I didn't need them to say anything, especially overzealous words about my future that sounded superficial."

—T.P., leukemia survivor

But when I got the call on my cell phone telling me I had cancer, the terror was physical; it was palpable as well as emotional. My heart pounded. I trembled.

Hearing the words, "It's cancer," terrified me more than anything I ever could have imagined.

"When you are diagnosed, when anyone's diagnosed with cancer, we cannot overestimate how vulnerable we become; how hard it is to think clearly; how anxiety distorts our sense, our judgment, our ability to think clearly," said therapist Halina Irving. "Whenever we face a terrible crisis, a terrible loss or a threat to our lives—trauma—we regress emotionally, and we need to be taken care of."

She continued, "Think of a child who has a trauma, whose mother goes away to the hospital for instance. A child who has given up the bottle asks for the bottle again; a child who has been toilet trained needs a diaper again. It's a temporary regression, but it has to do with the trauma of a diagnosis that robs us of the false sense of safety that we had that there was a future."

People who have cancer become more sensitive and vulnerable, especially soon after diagnosis, even if they seem to be in shock. "What cancer patients face is this other dimension of reality in which we have this constant awareness that we may not be able to go on living," said Irving.

"It's like being chased by a tiger in the woods. That's what it feels like."

Real and imagined fears

Remember being a child? When you were afraid, every shadow seemed to hide a monster. A creaking floorboard could conjure a vision of evil. Your heart jumped; your adrenaline coursed; you were ready to fight or fly the coop.

My adult family had been planning to fly our urban coop for the country for almost a year. Twice, in the autumn and spring, David and I had driven the ninety miles from our home to the small resort town of Guerneville to look at different vacation homes to rent with our best friends from Oregon. For the first time, they were coming to the Bay Area for our annual summer getaway; the past four years we'd traveled to the Oregon coast. We feared their sticker shock—everything in California seems to cost twice as much as in Oregon—and we wanted to find a place that was both economical and worth the drive down here.

I imagined our annual getaway sometimes with giddy excitement, other times with deep and spiritual serenity. How I looked forward to a week without makeup or pretense of any kind—long, wristwatch-free walks through the ancient redwoods, no pressure to make any decision except which pleasures to enjoy.

This summer we would treasure the hot sand-and-pebble beaches of the Russian River beneath our feet. Although the river itself would be quiet this time of year, we looked forward to hearing the laughter of children and teens inner-tubing in the clear green water and riding the Octopus and Ferris wheel at the amusement park nearby.

But just four days before our planned vacation, I received the news that I had cancer. While I was awaiting my diagnosis—technicians had been probing, piercing, scanning, and otherwise testing and taking biopsies of my tissues for almost a month —I learned that I would not have surgery for at least two or three weeks.

So I decided we would still take our vacation. I was looking forward to it like never before.

My best friend, Barbara, ranks among the most caring and compassionate people on the planet, and I needed compassion like I needed the breath that had been punched out of me earlier that week. I could hardly wait to see her. I knew she would listen to me and that her keen intelligence, sensitivity, and wisdom would soothe me. (I had no idea she would treat me to a deeply relaxing and much-needed massage to boot!)

"The word cancer scared me at first because I was dealing with the unknown, and I needed knowledge and encouragement."

—B.S., lymphoma survivor

When I mentioned to Angela, another friend, that I would be leaving the following Saturday for my family's annual vacation with our Oregon pals, she asked, "Do you think you'll be able to relax, knowing you have cancer and have to go in for surgery soon?"

"Oh, I'm sure I will," I assured her. I had recently begun to meditate, and I knew I would be able to relax in the towering pine and eucalyptus-scented forests.

I explained to Angela why I was so eager to get away, and she nodded and looked down. After a few moments of silence during which the refrigerator buzz grew as loud as a mosquito in my ear, the conversation moved on to something else.

Even though the conversation had moved on, her question remained in my mind, and I felt dizzy. Upset. Angry. Scared. Confused. "Why did she have to ask me that?" I wondered. "Why did she have to plant that awful seed of fear and doubt?"

The angel on my left shoulder assured me that she meant no harm. "It was just a question. Don't be so sensitive!" Those words, which I had heard many times in my youth, pulled my attention to the demon on my right shoulder.

It perched there, clouding my thoughts like thick, gray poison. "You *will* have an awful time. Angela is absolutely right. Why don't you postpone the trip? You'll probably have to come home midweek anyway for some medical test."

I thought I was losing my mind. How could one simple question hit me like a crowbar in the head? How did those few words make me a whirling dervish of good versus evil, faith versus fear?

I went on the trip, and though my nerve endings felt naked, my friends and family sheltered me with their love. I did have to drive back into town midweek to get a bone scan, but having Barbara and David along, both on the drive there and during the scan itself, served as an anesthetic to the psychic pain I feared I could not endure.

Though my fear did not dissipate, it was lessened by their love.

Fear of the simplest question: How are you?

It's not only words that have charged meanings when you have cancer; intonations can wield just as much power. Sometimes the way you say something can sound normal to you, the speaker, but the listener may hear it quite differently, causing him or her fear and anxiety.

For instance, take the simple question, "How are you?"

To a cancer patient or survivor, this off-the-cuff question we ask and answer dozens of times daily can cause pain, irritation, embarrassment, trepidation, or even shame.

Dr. Wendy Harpham, a physician, non-Hodgkin's lymphoma survivor, and author of three books about cancer, wrote an essay published in *Cure* magazine, "Surviving the Question: How ARE You?" She wrote:

"When I was first diagnosed with cancer, everyone asked me, 'How are you?' As if troops were gathering to wage battle against my fear and loneliness, 'How are you?' became a comforting code word for 'I'm on your side.' But within a few weeks, the chemotherapy began to take its toll, the shock and novelty of being a patient wore off, and I came to dread being asked, 'How are you?' This question undermined the distraction and healthy denial that minimized my distress . . . I found myself consoling those who asked, and then fighting the contagion of grief and fear."

"Suddenly, you're a mere mortal, and the possibility of death is real. There is also a sense of betrayal . . . how could my body give out on me this way?"

—J.J., uterine cancer survivor

Asking "How are you?" can mean many different things to a patient. Depending on the questioner's tone of voice, body language, rapport, level of intimacy and, of course, timing, it can gently soothe a soul, inflict pain, or awaken a sleeping fear.

Instead of asking an open-ended question about someone's state of being, a more benign way of inquiring might be to make the question more specific. Cancer survivor and oncology nurse Sandy Bezet trains the interns in her office to ask patients, "How are you *today*?" (my emphasis, not Bezet's) because, if someone asks, "How are you?" a patient's impulse may be to answer, "'How do you think I am?! I've been diagnosed with cancer!"

"Asking 'How are you today?' lets people know you really want to know how they are feeling today," said Bezet, "and I find patients are more likely to open up."

Bezet had just watched the film *Wit*— the movie version of Margaret Edson's Pulitzer Prize-winning Broadway play—with one of her interns. It tells the story of a brilliant, strong independent university professor dying of ovarian cancer, who talks about how often she is asked in the hospital how she is doing.

"I wonder if they'll ask me even as I'm dying," the professor wonders, and sure enough, they do. "'I'm fine, fine, fine,'" said Bezet. "It just became rote for her to say 'fine' because she realized that's what they needed to hear."

"How are you?" can also sound condescending, as can other expressions, said Bezet, like "when people lean over and tell you that they're sorry, and they pat you on the knee and say it with a little whisper, as if they're in the funeral home. Look me in the eye and say it, and say it in your regular voice as though I'm a living, breathing person who still has hobbies, has other interests beside this fear of dying!"

After Bezet was diagnosed with cancer, one of her patients came in crying because an innocent remark someone had made crushed her emotionally. Bezet told her boss, and he suggested they conduct a survey of patients to see which remarks helped and which didn't.

"We put three-by-five cards at the appointment desk," Bezet said, "asking people to write down the right thing to say and the wrong thing to say. Sometimes the things written on the 'right things to say' lists are the same as those written on the 'wrong things to say' list, but we came up with a list that a lot of patients agreed on."

Bezet was generous and shared the list, and many of the comments appear throughout this book. But, again, what's important in choosing words is putting yourself in the other person's place.

For example, "How aaarrreeee you?" asked of a person who finished treatment six months ago may take them back to a place they'd just managed to escape. Sometimes when people ask me "How aaarrreeee you?" it's like falling asleep and hearing the phone ring—the question harkens back to a time filled with dangers and warnings. That's because it is difficult to forget you had cancer, and sometimes you just want to put and *keep* it out of your mind.

In my case, I like people to ask me how I am doing in a casual way, as in, "How you doin'?" If I feel like sharing my fear about an imminent CT scan or a dream about my cancer recurring, well, they asked for it. If not, I'm free to converse like a normal person—instead of a tumor with arms, legs, a body, and a head.

Fear of treatment and its effects

Johanna Endreson had just earned her master's degree in public policy when her boyfriend, Martin, proposed to her on a Hawaiian vacation. It was August 2001; they set a wedding date almost a year in advance to make sure their nuptials fit their dreams.

"We had done a lot of planning for it. And then in February, I felt a lump in my neck," Johanna told me over coffee one morning at a café across the street from the University of California at Berkeley. "I wasn't actually thinking it was anything like cancer and didn't feel even remotely worried, but I wanted to get out of work, so I went to see the doctor."

The doctor told her not to worry, that it was probably a swollen gland. But a month later, Johanna felt another lump and went back to the doctor. During the next few weeks, she underwent an extensive series of tests and biopsies.

"In the beginning of April, we got the biopsy results, and he said I had stage three Hodgkin's disease and that I would have to do twelve weeks of chemo and four weeks of radiation."

The cancer had spread to her neck, chest, and spleen. The doctors told her she could lose her fertility and that there was no time to save any of her eggs before starting treatment, because it would require two cycles of menstruation.

Johanna was shocked, terrified, and horribly disappointed. She realized she would be just finishing up her twelve-week round of chemo on her wedding day.

"A couple of days after my diagnosis, Martin said, 'What are we going to do, wait until July?'"

Johanna was supposed to start treatment in three weeks. But she and Martin decided to get married the week before her chemo. That gave them two weeks to prepare.

"So we planned a wedding," Johanna laughed. "We had seventy people show up. And the thing that was amazing was that so many people came and helped us with things. Martin's aunt bought my dress. A florist gave us a discount because she was moved by what was going on. One of my best friends just called everyone and said, 'Okay, Johanna's having her wedding; come on!' My employer even let us use my work building for the reception."

"Please know that we are scared, and for someone who lives alone just a simple hug can fill us more than a great dinner out. They say of the five senses, deprivation of touch is the most severe. A hug or holding of one's hand can release the fears and allow ourselves to feel cared about."

—D.K., melanoma survivor

The wedding was beautiful. Nine days later she started chemotherapy.

"That day, I cut off all my hair, just so when it fell out, I wouldn't have to have it bald long."

Cutting her hair off was almost more frightening than anything else she went through. Her well-meaning friends didn't make it any easier.

Johanna had the kind of hair that turned heads half a block away. Long, black, and curly, it was the product of an aesthetically gorgeous blending of cultures; her mother is Italian, and her father is African American. The hair she had worn long for more years than she could remember had grown past her slender waist.

But losing what she had always considered her most beautiful physical gift and a central part of her identity—her hair—was causing her intense fear.

"I think within the African American community, especially for women, there's a big emphasis on our hair. So when I found out that I had cancer, that was the thing a lot of black women I knew related to. The first thing they would say was, 'Oooooh, you're going to lose your hair? But you have such good hair!' or 'Oh, that's horrible!'"

What made it so frightening for Johanna was not only that her hair would fall out, but that it was something totally out of her control.

"The doctor said, 'You might become infertile; you might have problems with this or that. But you're definitely going to lose your hair.' I could have hope about everything else, but I knew I was definitely going to lose my hair."

Johanna said two camps of people tried to help her cope with her imminent loss, but both ended up taking her to a place she didn't feel ready to go.

"There were people who were 'awfulizing' it—who made losing my hair feel like the end of the world and the worst possible thing. And there were other people who trivialized it, like, 'Why are you being so vain? Why do you even care about this? I mean, that's the least of your concerns.'"

Johanna knew Martin cherished her hair too. He couldn't watch the haircut, so he dropped her off at the salon. But the words he spoke upon seeing her new do were the perfect ones.

"'Oh, my God, you're so much prettier with short hair! Oh, my God, I love it!' he told me. He was so sweet!"

Johanna remains positive about her experience. Although she feels she was a happy person before her cancer, she feels stronger now in many ways. Battling cancer gave her the courage to do things she never would have felt confident enough to do before.

"I never would have gone back to get my PhD," she said thoughtfully. "There's never been a black person in the public policy doctoral program, and there have only been thirty-three PhDs in that program ever. I think I would have been way too scared, but now I'm not. I can do chemo. And radiation was in some ways worse than the chemo. So I can do a PhD!"

Fear can prevent all of us from taking risks, and when you have cancer, fighting for your life can seem like a huge risk. Acknowledging cancer patients' fears, without fueling them, can help them live through their terror.

Loaded words

Some words and phrases almost automatically induce anxiety. Words like *mortality rate* and *recurrence* have implications that can trip up a cancer patient or survivor as surely as a stone in the road.

Harvard psychology professor Ellen Langer wrote about a word that carries immense weight: *remission*. And she should know. Her mother died of breast cancer at fifty-six, but before that, the medical profession had declared that her mother's disease had gone into "complete remission."

In an essay published in *Psychology Today,* Langer questioned what that label means.

"If two people go for a checkup to see if they have cancer and one never had the disease while the other person is in 'remission,' the test results look the same," she wrote. "Psychologically, however, 'remission' may be very different from a 'cure.' Language has the interesting property of being able to increase and decrease our perception of control. Different word choices can direct our thoughts about a single situation in many different ways.

"Consider the way we deal with cancer. If somebody has cancer and the cancer goes away, we say it is in remission. The implication is that the same cancer will recur."

I remember the first time someone asked me whether my cancer was in remission. My stomach sank, as if I had suddenly flown into turbulent skies. It was soon after my surgery, and it hadn't occurred to me that I might have to go under the knife again anytime in my lifetime. I had been so focused on my treatment and on the test results that showed the cancer hadn't spread to my lymph nodes that I had not allowed myself to imagine that I might have to hear "You have cancer" ever again.

Langer wondered whether the word *remission* contributed to her mother's death.

"Being in remission means that we are waiting for 'it' to return. . . Psychologically, this may lead us to feel defeated. For each new cold we beat, we implicitly think, 'I beat it before, I can beat it again.' If the cancer comes back, however, we think, 'It is winning. I am just not as strong as it is. . . .

"It is clear that giving up impairs people's physical health and keeps them from wanting to survive. Why exercise or take medication if one is likely to die soon anyway? Did cancer kill my mother, or was it the language that we used to describe cancer that led her to give up?"

Most of the time, it's not a matter of life and death, of course, but certain words can shape our perceptions. One relative asked me how I was "progressing" after my surgery. To me, diseases "progress," whereas health "improves." Another person asked if I was "maintaining." To me, "maintaining" implies an imminent drop, as in airspeed. When I read in an obituary that an acquaintance, beloved journalist Faith Fancher, had "succumbed" to cancer, it angered me, because *succumb* implies that that she gave up and allowed the cancer to win. Perhaps she did surrender to death—we must all surrender our lives, after all—but she had a fighting spirit, and I don't think she would have liked anyone implying that she submitted to the disease itself, that she gave up and gave in. I believe she died fighting.

Though subtle, these linguistic differences enlarge under the magnifying glass of illness. But that doesn't mean that someone necessarily will ignite under such a lens. And if a flame does erupt, it can be extinguished with tenderness and understanding.

Sometimes it's better to keep your words to yourself; instead, open your ears and your heart. Allowing your loved one to express his or her fears—without trying to assuage them—can be the greatest life-giver of all.

5.
"I need you to listen to me and let me cry."

Remember that silence is sometimes the best answer.

—The Dalai Lama

"KEEP YOUR EYES AND EARS OPEN AND YOUR MOUTH SHUT!" He moved his mouth with the speed and precision of a karate master's kick, shocking, disarming, and terrifying his young charges. His cold blue eyes stayed focused as they sliced through the boys like a fighter jet through clouds.

Although none were yet twenty years old, the boys—some gangly, some shaped like the McNuggets they had lived on—looked like men in their uniform blue prison garb. Their faces registered sheepishness, fear, and shame, as if they had just gotten their first haircuts. Most *had* just gotten their first buzz cut. Robbed of their lovely locks, they may have felt like post-chemo cancer patients. But these boys were being punished, losing their ponytails and mullet cuts as partial payment for their transgressions.

It was the '80s, and I was making a documentary about prison overcrowding. We traveled to Georgia to visit a boot camp to see how teens who had violated the law were being discouraged from doing so again as adults, when the stakes would be much higher.

My photographer, Steve, captured the moment beautifully on videotape. And though I can remember little of the documentary, I cannot get those words out of my mind: "Keep your eyes and ears open and your mouth shut!"

As the buzz-topped corporal told me later in his molasses drawl, "It sure gets their attention." It sure did, especially since they had to drop and do one hundred push-ups if they failed to comply. Most of us don't live with that kind of threat. So how do we learn to keep our eyes and ears open and our mouths shut—in other words, how do we learn to listen?

Telling it like it is

For an answer, I turned to Jeff Kane, MD. I had just read what I consider his masterpiece of compassion, *How to Heal: A Guide for Caregivers*. I am awed at his ability to communicate so clearly the nuts and bolts of caregiving, which comes down to, basically, listening.

"Keep your eyes and ears open and your mouth shut!" Again, those words echo in my mind. Kane delivers the same message in his book, but he whispers it gently, and with great love, transforming the demand into a polite request, a simple plea that makes one eager to comply.

I drove almost four hours across the hay-colored Sacramento Valley and through the Sierra Nevada Mountains to spend just twice as many hours with this man and the individuals he accompanies through their private hells.

I felt like *I* had entered hell as I opened my car door, grabbed my briefcase, and walked through the baking parking lot of Sierra Nevada Cancer Center in Grass Valley, California. I could feel the heat of the pavement through my shoes. Although it was October, it was as hot and dry as August; though Grass Valley is relatively close to the temperate Bay Area, it seemed as if I was worlds away.

Dr. Kane was about to lead a cancer support group, and I was to meet with him beforehand. I made my way to the stark meeting room, and within a few minutes, I saw a tall man with tightly curled hair speckled black and gray like river rocks walk into the room. He offered me a kind smile that revealed great vulnerability.

We had barely ten minutes to talk before the members of the support group started dribbling into the room, which was crowded by a large, square featureless Formica table. Lit by cool fluorescent lights, the space rendered all complexions pink and blue.

Greetings were made, and soon the table twittered with conversation and the emotional timbre rose.

"Okay, let's check in," Dr. Kane interrupted, volume raised just enough to get their attention.

After introducing me—he didn't need to ask the group's permission for me to attend, since I'm a cancer survivor myself—he turned his gaze, head slightly tilted, to each of the eight men and women around the table. When he looked at them, you got the sense that it was just him and his pals at a kitchen table.

"How have the last couple of weeks been?"

Harold, a man to my right who is two heads taller than me sitting down, warmed the room with his baritone bellow and flame-red hair; he's a friendly giant, with a jolly voice to match.

"Doing okay," he said. A long pause.

Dr. Kane lowered his chin to catch Harold's downcast eyes. "How's your family situation?" Dr. Kane and the group knew Harold's sister had recently died of cancer, and they suspected it had brought up fears and anger forgotten in the eight years since his own cancer diagnosis.

"I never felt that people were 'hurtful,' but I did get the impression that a lot of the time they didn't want to hear about how sick or tired I was feeling from chemo.... I didn't expect them to do anything about my nausea or fatigue, I just wanted them to listen and understand."

—A.D., breast cancer survivor

"I ignore everything on both sides," Harold laughed, referring to certain members of his family that he does not get along with. More silence. "I gave up on them a long time ago." More silence as Harold considered what he needed to say next.

Harold's own cancer nightmare began after an X-ray revealed a mass in his lung. After the fourth attempt to biopsy the nodule, his lung collapsed. As surely as the needle deflated his lung, the words "You have cancer" left him breathless.

No one looked away from Harold as he explained a recent visit to his dermatologist to check out a rash on his shoulder. "My thoughts immediately went to cancer."

Heads around the table bobbed subtly with affirmation. When you've had cancer, each bump, each lump, every headache can be a harbinger of cells run amuck, even years later.

Harold told the story. The dermatologist examined the rash, then he noticed Harold's midsection. He asked what the scar was from, and Harold told him he had had a lobectomy; that he had had cancer.

"Well, this rash is harmless," the doctor declared. "You're not paranoid, are you?"

Harold shook his head. "So I told him, 'You get lung cancer and see what it does to your paranoia level!'"

Everyone in the group laughed, recalling their own hangnail-turned-tumor story.

"That's what I love about coming here," Harold said, looking fondly from face to face. "I can tell you when my fingers have been bothering me, and no one gets upset. My wife does, though."

"Cancer patients are aware of the fact that cancer does have a tendency to come back. When the patient verbalizes this fear, don't minimize it or trivialize it. Be supportive."

—J.K., lung cancer survivor

The group members loved being able to say, with impunity, whatever they wanted. They didn't have to worry about worrying their spouses with their "paranoia"; they could laugh at one another's fears, knowing the fears would pass.

Dr. Kane went around the room, checking in with the other members, many of whom he had known for several years.

Mitchell, a gastroenterologist, told the group he might not be seeing them for a while since he would be flying to Boston every month for an experimental cancer treatment involving a new drug. "My eight-by-ten-centimeter mass will be removed first," he explained clinically, adding in a much softer voice, "I met a woman on the Internet who has the same thing; the drug didn't work for her after one year."

No one said a word. They didn't tell him everything would be okay. They just listened, allowing him to express himself.

Opening an oyster

Over coffee later, Dr. Kane explained that his support groups work because they not only facilitate listening, they acknowledge suffering.

"Part of the skill is just recognizing that [as the listener] you are experiencing pain. You're absorbing pain from this other person, but it's not going to damage you. It's not like you have your hand in a fire. It won't damage you as long as you recognize it, inhale, drink it in, and then exhale it out—let it go."

Everyone needs to acknowledge and release their pain, said Dr. Kane. "You just get it out, drain the abscess, and finally, you're at acceptance. And that's when the work starts."

"You're like a therapist in your support group," I observed, "even though you're considered a facilitator."

"You can think of it as therapy. But I really think of it as friendship. How would a friend behave with you? A real friend. A real friend would draw out your feelings."

I commented on how enlightened Dr. Kane seemed to be. It amazed me that he had a following of people ranging from a cabinetmaker to a doctor to a sixty-eight-year-old near-hermit who was given a year and a half to live eight years ago. These oldsters were not New Agers.

"These people are standard white middle-class folks," Dr. Kane laughed. "They don't know from meditation or therapy or anything. I don't have a contract with them. Their doctors say, 'Go to the support group.' That means a lot of people whining to each other, as far as they know."

"I wanted to have my feelings acknowledged and accepted."

—D.W., colon cancer survivor

Dr. Kane probes them gently, at first. Not everyone feels comfortable in the group, so he talks about how unusual this kind of conversation is. He encourages them to talk about that and then, if they are ready, to talk about themselves.

He asks them, "How is it for you?" Sometimes they answer with vague, tentative responses, and he asks them to tell him more. As they relax and talk more, they sometimes share things they haven't told anyone before.

"You know Anne Lamott, who writes about writing in *Bird by Bird*? It's what she calls 'the really shitty first draft.' They just blurt something out. It's something they don't want to say or may have never said. They're uncomfortable saying it. They're not really familiar with what they're say-ing. And you listen well enough to allow them to say it.

"Like their first draft might be anger at you. They don't really mean that. But it's anger and you're handy. And so you can stay around and say to them, 'What's that like?' 'You're a rotten son of a bitch, really,' they might say. 'Tell me more about that,' I say. And they just go on."

One thing Dr. Kane asks each group member is what bothers him or her about having cancer. That can anger some people, but when they follow the conversation to its logical end, it usually helps. Although it can take a while to figure it out, most conclude, "It means I'm going to die."

"Okay, so what's new about that? I could have told you you're going to die," Kane tells them. He then asks what bothers them about dying? They begin to think about it. "Well, I have business to finish," they might say. "Really? What sort of business?" Kane might ask. And they think about it. One cancer patient said, "Well, I want to reconcile with my kids."

"What's really bothering this woman about her cancer is the cancer's telling her she might die with unfinished business," Kane explained. And now she knows what it is. And she knows what to do about it. There's nothing I need to do. I can't tell her. I can't interpret. My role is just to ask the questions that lead her into the center of it."

Hold my hand

"Where did you come from?" I asked Dr. Kane. Although I knew he prac-ticed medicine as an emergency room physician in Berkeley for ten years before learning how to heal as opposed to "cure" people, I couldn't under-stand how he got from there to here. He sees it as an act of grace.

"I just went into the ER one day, and I was dissatisfied with it. . . . It felt like I'd been trained to be an engineer—that I was just operating a turn-stile—people come in and I fix them and kick them out again. I wasn't sure what my values were; all I knew was that it didn't feel right."

Dr. Kane quit his job and never looked back. He ended up teaching phi-losophy at a community college, then he became a yoga teacher. But he returned to conventional medicine as a healer: He founded the support pro-grams at Sacramento's Sutter Cancer Center and Grass Valley's Sierra Nevada Cancer Center, later becoming the director of psychosocial educa-tion and ultimately winning the Health Communication Research Institute's "Heroes in Healthcare" Lifetime Achievement Award. He has been leading support groups for almost three decades and frequently speaks to physicians' and other caregivers' groups around the nation.

Still the philosopher, Dr. Kane explained why he sees himself as a friend rather than as a therapist.

"The model I use is Virgil and Dante." He was referring to the *Inferno*, the *Divine Comedy*'s story of the trip to Hell. "The illustrations always show Virgil holding Dante's hand—always, in every picture, leading him to Hell. Dante's always horrified, confused, enraged, and frightened. And each time, Virgil is just there holding his hand, encouraging him, supporting him.

> *"Allow your friend to say how they are really feeling and don't feel that you have to 'fix it.' Listening is enough."*
>
> —S.B., cervical cancer survivor

"It's different than the healing of the doctor-patient relationship, which is more vertical. It's just being human—and not having to fix it."

Asking questions and listening to answers seemed to come easily to Dr. Kane. But he admitted that he still struggles to be a friend. As a trained physician, he sometimes finds himself wanting to ask what a patient needs, even when he knows that will not be productive. He suspects it is because he wants to stop them from talking, because they're telling him about their pain at a time when he has had enough.

Dr. Kane said that what usually helps someone most has little to do with words or actions. "What everyone tells me is that as soon as they get diagnosed, all this stuff begins to accumulate next to their bed: books, diets, crystals. The stuff just comes. This notion that you can help by giving something is noble. It sounds altruistic, but it doesn't work. What really helps is to *bring something out of the person*: 'Tell me how you're suffering.'"

Crying out

I'll never forget the first time I saw my father cry. I think I was five or six. We were having breakfast at our glossy red 1950s-style glass-topped kitchen table. Dad was always so cheerful in the morning, and I recall him reaching for the *St. Louis Globe Democrat* with a wide smile that disappeared in an instant as he knocked his boiling cup of instant Folgers coffee into his lap.

"Oh, my God!" my mother screamed, popping out of her chair like toast. She ran to the freezer to grab some ice.

Dad didn't scream, but his eyes scrunched up and filled with tears and his face wrinkled in a mask of agony. I started crying, too.

"It was difficult for me to hear from my husband that I need to stop feeling sorry for myself at times when I was depressed or needed to cry."

—M.M., breast cancer survivor

"It's okay," Mom cooed. "Daddy just has an owie. He'll be okay. You just go into your room, darling," she said. She turned to me, leaving the freezer open, and gave me a temporary pink lipstick tattoo on my forehead. She hugged me and led me by hand into the room she had painted herself with teddy bears and bunny rabbit appliqués.

But they were no comfort; I was panicked and confused and sat motionless on my bed. A few minutes later I heard my parents laughing in the kitchen; they were probably trying to figure out how to explain to me what had happened. No explanation was necessary. I knew all I needed to know: "Daddy was okay!" And, "Daddy can cry!"

My next experience seeing a grownup in tears was almost more shocking and at least as terrifying.

The school principal came to our classroom and beckoned our teacher, Mrs. Coffey, into the hall. When Mrs. Coffrey returned, head bowed and silent, oblivious to the chatter of fifth-graders, we looked at her, puzzled. Forty little eyes saw something that challenged their idea of reality: a teacher transformed by tears into a human being.

"Boys and girls," she said, pausing to suppress her tears so she could speak, "President Kennedy has been shot." She began to weep.

Adults everywhere cried unashamedly that day, and for the first time, children could witness a flood of tears on television. We silently asked ourselves, "How can we be safe with so many grownups crying? Who will protect us?"

There was one leader I knew would shelter us from harm: Jackie Kennedy. She didn't cry.

"First Lady Holds Strong for Nation," read the headlines.

I do remember puzzling over how she could control her tears. It seemed so odd to me that anyone could keep up such a strong front if she were really suffering. Surely she must have ached deeply enough to shed tears. But she never did cry, at least as far as I knew. She was a model of strength, a dignified pillar supporting a colonial structure of immeasurable beauty; she symbolized our nation's fortitude in the face of fear or foe.

Forty years later, almost to the day, another headline about the Kennedy family shattered my sense of reality: "Diary Reveals Grief of Jackie Kennedy."

An Associated Press article reported the story: "To a grieving nation, Jacqueline Kennedy was stoic after her husband's assassination. But over games of tennis with a priest who counseled her, she apparently revealed her feelings, including thoughts of suicide."

"I'm so bleeding inside," she had told Rev. Richard McSorley, who had recently died, leaving behind his typewritten diary which included recollections of his private conversations with Mrs. Kennedy.

The Associated Press article continued, "The release has raised questions about the propriety of a priest keeping notes on private discussions." But to me, it raised questions about hiding one's feelings—about keeping a stiff upper lip and sucking it up. I was relieved that Mrs. Kennedy had not only experienced but also had expressed her grief, at least to one person.

Six months after the assassination, she had written McSorley saying she would never get over her loss. But what if she had revealed her grief? What if she had talked about her feelings of dread, hopelessness, and fear? Would that have made it easier for her to recover from her loss?

Telling your story makes it real

Like Jackie Kennedy, Ruth Redford loves tennis. In fact, that's how I learned of her, through a friend who belongs to the same tennis club on Harbor Bay, an island of suburban charm on the San Francisco Bay.

Ruth is not one for just small talk at the club. She is a lover of the mind as well as the body. After working as a physical therapist for almost a quarter century, she recently earned a master's degree in philosophy.

"People think philosophy is so esoteric, but to me, philosophy is everything," she said. No need to convince me of that. I earned a BA in philosophy, and to this day I still "love the questions themselves, like locked doors," as Rainer Maria Rilke advised in Letters to a Young Poet.

Ruth continued. "Philosophy comes down to the very core of what you think about yourself as a human being and how you relate to fellow human beings; to me, that is the most integral thing there can possibly be in your life."

But one thing is even more essential: life itself. Ruth realized that when her sister was diagnosed with breast cancer.

"She had a horrendous, horrendous time," Ruth began. "They originally thought it was DCIS [ductile carcinoma in situ, which means precancerous cells], and they said it was no big deal."

But when surgeons operated on Ruth's sister, they found other tumors that hadn't been picked up on the mammogram, so she ended up having a mastectomy. The cancer had spread to her lymph nodes, and she had to undergo surgery again, which resulted in an infection that required a week's hospitalization. Finally, she had breast reconstructive surgery.

You can imagine Ruth's fear when she felt a lump in her own breast one year later. An ultrasound showed nothing, so Ruth didn't let herself worry about it any more. But four months later, when she went in for her regular gynecological checkup, the lump was still palpable.

A fine needle biopsy was inconclusive, so she had another mammogram, an ultrasound, and ultimately a core biopsy. That's when she was diagnosed with cancer.

"But the odd thing is—and the reason I tell this whole story—is that what they found is not the lump we originally felt," Ruth said excitedly. "My malignancy was very small, very deep, almost on the chest wall. The radiologist could hardly find it. So in a lot of ways, I was very lucky. And I feel like I sort of have my sister to thank for it, because it was her having the cancer that put up the red flag that they had to be extra cautious with me."

Although finding the tumor was a relief, Ruth feared she faced the same outcome as her sister.

"But my doctor kept saying to me, 'Ruth, you're not your sister. You're not your sister.'"

When they went in to remove it, the tumor was twice as large as they had gathered from viewing the mammogram and ultrasound. But Ruth would not require more surgery, and she would have to undergo only radiation, not chemotherapy. She had just begun radiation treatment when we spoke.

"I'll just go on with life as usual. If I have to deal with something, I will."

But she was more philosophical when she spoke about the experience of being diagnosed.

"It's a very surreal experience being diagnosed with cancer. You feel totally normal, and all of a sudden somebody's saying you have this very potentially life-threatening thing.

"For me, it was more of a psychological adjustment. After a week or so, it was almost like I was shell-shocked, and my tendency was just to go home and let it kind of filter in." But she realized what she needed to do was talk about it.

"Sometimes someone would ask how I was, and when we started talking cancer, they changed the subject. That made me feel horrible."

—M.L., breast cancer survivor

"I was reading this one article for a philosophy class, and what this person was writing was that the boundary between the real and the unreal is much more blurred than what we would, in a normal sense, or intellectually, want to countenance. It talked about how important the narrative is—that is, the storytelling. That's what makes something real."

Ruth explained that she needed to tell the story of her cancer diagnosis to people in order to believe it herself.

"It was really important for me to talk about it over and over again because that's what made it real. It was like the talking about it somehow allowed me psychologically to let it become a part of my reality. And I started thinking about it, and I realized that I've experienced that throughout my life. I remember when I got engaged. It didn't seem real until I told people about it. Or when I was pregnant. They tell you you're pregnant, but you don't really feel it in your body, so it's not real until you talk about it and draw other people into that reality with you. Then it becomes part of your life history or part of your life narrative."

Ruth said cancer was beginning to feel more like her history than her present, partly because of a conversation she had with her radiation nurse the day before.

"She was giving me all these handouts. And one was put out by the American Cancer Society. It was a list of resources for people with cancer. And the nurse said to me, 'Well, this doesn't really apply to you because you no longer have cancer, and what we're doing now is preventive.'"

Ruth let out a deep breath. "That was like a whole different way of thinking about it, all of a sudden just to say, you know, it's gone! Not even like I'm in remission. And I know, intellectually, the purpose of radiation is, if there are still cells in there, to kill the cells. But at the same time, it was like a different way of looking at my reality.

"My husband felt he had to be 'the man' and not get emotional. I needed him to cry with me and to understand how afraid I was—and to let me have that feeling. Ultimately, I had to understand that it was probably too much for him, especially after losing his father so soon before my own diagnosis."

—B.G., breast cancer survivor

"But back to when I was first diagnosed," Ruth continued, eager to return to the meaning of her diagnosis. "It was painful for me to talk about it, but I also realized it was therapeutic for me to talk about it. And once you do, it somehow doesn't seem quite as scary."

The problem was, some of her friends didn't welcome conversation about her cancer.

"They wanted to express support, but they were also afraid that they were going to make me sad. And so it would be sort of like, 'Let's not talk about it because I don't want to make you sad.' That kind of thing. And, 'Let's just do something happier.' And I certainly wanted to go out and still laugh and have fun with my friends, but I think people should know it's okay to talk about it and it's okay if I cry, because those things all help me get through the process."

But sometimes when Ruth cried, it made her feel worse.

"As soon as you start crying, people think they're making it more painful for you instead of helping you work through it. But for me, to verbalize things is to make them not only more real but less threatening. Because when you're holding it all inside and working it over in your mind again and again, it becomes ten times worse."

It made me wonder what it was like for Jackie Kennedy. As a nation, being able to release our tears collectively helped us cope with the assassination of her husband, one of our greatest leaders. We talked about his loss for weeks, months, and years; most of us who were alive at the time can remember exactly where we were that day. It became part of the national narrative, and talking about it helped us heal.

President John F. Kennedy was known for his call, "Ask not what your country can do for you, but what you can do for your country." Now is the time, when your friend or loved one has cancer, to ask what you can do for her or him. And that means listening.

How to listen

Dolores Moorehead directs a program at the Women's Cancer Resource Center (WCRC) in Oakland, a nonprofit organization that provides information and support at no charge to all women throughout the San Francisco Bay Area who are impacted by cancer. The organization sponsors numerous support groups (including a posttreatment group I attend), and it gets hundreds of calls weekly requesting information and referral services. Often, the callers just need to talk. It's imperative that the WCRC workers know how to listen.

Students from the University of California at Berkeley often intern at WCRC to earn credit toward their degrees. Moorehead trains them to answer the phones.

"A lot of them are very concerned about saying the wrong thing. And my feeling is that you can't say the wrong thing," Moorehead explained. She said people sometimes say less-than-ideal things because they become uncomfortable with silence. "But if you're a really good listener, you listen, and the silence is okay."

Moorehead said when we fill in the silence, we tend to speak without thinking, and sometimes something inappropriate comes out. She advises her interns, "You listen to the person; you allow them to have their silence. And you think before you respond. It doesn't mean you know the answers."

Like Dr. Jeff Kane, Moorehead believes that problems often arise because someone wants to solve a problem, so they provide a fix-it answer. But women who call WCRC are not necessarily looking for answers, just for someone who will listen with an open heart and mind. They need someone on the end of the line who will keep their ears open and their mouth shut.

Obviously, one cannot keep one's mouth shut continuously, and it is important that the person with cancer knows that he or she is being heard. Many therapists and communications professionals recommend "mirroring," or reflecting back to the person what they just said, not word for word, but by paraphrasing their meaning.

For example, if someone tells you they are afraid, rather than urging them not to be fearful, you can simply acknowledge their feelings by saying something like, "It is scary," or "That sounds frightening."

You can also listen well by clarifying what the speaker has said to you. In other words, if they say, "I don't want to go back to the doctor tomorrow," you might respond, "It sounds like you're saying the doctor makes you feel uncomfortable." That way it opens the door and encourages the person to express rather than repress his or her feelings.

Though people with cancer do need someone to listen, they also need to listen to others, and sometimes they may even welcome hearing about other people's problems, since it takes their mind off of their own. But it's a good idea to ask permission before heaping your troubles upon someone who has cancer. It's a good idea, in fact, to ask permission before doing a lot of things for, or saying a lot of things to, someone with cancer.

6.

"Asking my permission
can spare me pain."

**It's easier to ask forgiveness than permission.
[But it can cause a lot more suffering.]**

—Anonymous

SUSAN CHERNAK MCELROY DRINKS A LOT. That's how she describes her-self to people, often those whom she has just met. Not only does she disarm folks with that statement, she ups the ante when she tells them why. Most don't know whether to laugh or cry.

Susan had cancer of the mouth, and most of her salivary glands have been surgically removed, so she has to sip liquids to keep her mouth hydrated.

She and I sipped coffee as I interviewed her just after breakfast in a low-lit dining room of a hotel with a forestlike atrium, complete with water-falls. Susan, a best-selling author and sought-after speaker, was presenting at a "Cancer as a Turning Point" conference across the street, and I was there searching for stories and inspiration. I had slipped Susan a note intro-ducing myself and requesting an interview the afternoon before at her book signing, but had not heard back from her. Serendipitously, I ran into her at the hotel buffet breakfast the next day. She greeted me like an old friend, though we hadn't exchanged any words, and soon her stories flowed easily.

When Susan discovered she had cancer, she had been working at a job as an environmental technical editor, which she loved—though not as much as working with animals. Unfortunately, her work with critters could not pay the rent, which is why she had embarked upon a new career, using a talent people had told her for years that she had—that of a writer. (And she is gifted, indeed: Her book *Animals as Teachers and Healers* was a *New York Times* best seller.)

"I was working with a wonderful firm when I discovered a lump under my tongue," Susan said, looking down and moving her fork back and forth in a little arc on the table. "After surgery and a round of chemotherapy, doctors told me I was just fine. But eight months later, it came back.

"The well of fear was so enormous," she recalled nervously, stopping the fork abruptly. "And I had been a person so easily swayed by the influence of others that I became intuitively aware very early on in the process that I needed to watch what was told to me."

Susan said she has always known how sensitive she is. "Other people's words have governed me my whole life. Am I okay? Does my boyfriend think I'm okay? Do my parents need me to be like that? Do the teachers want me to be like this? Then all of a sudden you've got cancer. And you think, Are they telling me to be dead? I'll be a good girl and be dead!'"

Often Susan was able to control what others said to her, including the dentist who first broke the news that her tumor was malignant. "I said, 'Don't tell me what kind it is. I'm not ready to hear it.' My dog had died of malignant melanoma, and I didn't want to hear the word 'melanoma' because she had a tumor in her mouth just like I did. And my dentist respected that."

"I didn't like having meals delivered unless I was asked on that day because some days I hated looking at or smelling food."

—M.D., breast cancer survivor

But not everyone respected or understood her sensitivity to words. After her tumor was removed, one young hospital resident she saw told her she had a 92 percent chance of recurrence within a year. "And he was saying, 'You're doing really well now, but we've really got to track you.' Well, why? 'Because you have blah blah blah.'"

Susan interrupted him and asked where he got the 92 percent figure.

"He said it was in all the statistical data. And I said, 'Yeah, but didn't you also just tell me that I'm probably the only woman my age with this in the entire county? So I don't fall into that statistical data, do I? So my case could be way better or way worse!' And he said, 'You know, I hadn't thought of that.'"

Susan warned the resident, "You watch that. Watch it, because I hear you. And new patients hear you."

After finishing her story, I felt like applauding, but instead I remarked that she is a great teacher.

"No, I'm just a bully," she laughed. "He was good, and he caught on."

Not everyone catches on to the idea of filtering what they say. The person who probably loves Susan more than anyone else on earth didn't seem to have a clue as to how much power her words wielded.

"Mom wanted me to come to her house and do my recuperation there. I had a sense that that would not work for me, that I needed to be alone . . . I did not need my mom's fear on top of me through that. But Mom wanted to take care of me. So she called me up one day and said, 'I really want you to come and stay with me and Dad.'"

Though Susan said she wanted to stay at her boyfriend's house, because he worked all day and she could enjoy some much-needed rest and solitude there, her mother insisted.

"I called your dentist up the other day," Susan's mom began. "He told me about cancers like yours; he told me that what will happen is that it will just keep coming back, and it will eat away your tongue and it will eat away your jaw and it will eat away your entire face and then you'll be dead. And will your boyfriend take care of you then?"

Susan sighed, making the arc again with her fork. But she smiled crookedly and looked up, eyes twinkling. "I said, 'Good-bye, Mom,' and I hung up the phone." Silence for a moment, then, "She has no memory of ever having said that. I think that catastrophic illness can bring the crazies out in people. And they'll blurt out their worst fears onto you."

Susan said her cancer created a well of fear for almost everyone around her. "I was almost expecting to take care of everyone else. I remember my mother once saying to me, sobbing on my shoulder, 'You have to tell me you'll be okay.' And I said, 'Mom, you're my mother. You're supposed to be telling *me* I'm going to be okay. So if you need to hear I'm going to be okay, you need to find it from someone other than me. Go talk to your friends and ask them to tell you.'"

"Asking" is a key word and concept for Susan. Few of us ask permission before dumping our feelings onto someone else. But that is particularly important when dealing with someone who has cancer—someone who may be at their very weakest and most vulnerable and can't support the weight of their own terror, much less someone else's.

Susan drew on her experience with animals, about which she has written extensively.

"Nature works by the law of consent and permission. Animals and trees don't spend their time running away from situations that aren't good. They spend their time using all of their senses to gravitate to what attracts them. If something does not attract them, they leave. If a seed tries to grow in a place where the sun is not consenting, it will die. The more consent you have in your life, the more you will thrive. That's how animals do well. It's not survival of the fittest. It's who has the most consent."

Susan said animals go to a place and watch to get a sense of whether it's safe. They get a sense of whether the water's clean, whether there's good food. They go where they are attracted. If animals step into a place in nature where they are not welcome, they will die. If they don't establish consent, Susan maintained, it could cost them their lives because they could miss the fact that a predator is waiting to pounce.

"Part of consent is asking permission," Susan observed, the intensity of her voice increasing as she pushed the fork to her right, almost off the table. "People don't ask permission for anything. I know that because I'm a real bullish person. But when I go into nature, if I ask consent to be there, if I ask if I'm welcome in this place, I start to feel a kind of yes or no. I realize how important that process is for thriving and living in balance."

Susan wished that, as a cancer patient, her friends and family had asked for her consent. "You know, like, 'Do you want to hear treatment options? I've been looking into this.' And I could have said yes or no. Or if they would have asked, 'Can I talk to you about my own fears?' I could have said, 'Not today.' Or, 'Yes, I would love to hear about them.'"

Susan said if people would just ask permission before bludgeoning cancer patients with their feelings, it would keep them from making stupid blunders. "It would keep them from saying stuff like, 'Oh, I knew somebody who had that and they're dead now.'"

Susan uses her own sensitivity and pain to try to spare other cancer patients the intense fear and discomfort she has experienced. When she meets someone who mentions they have had cancer, she assumes they are newly diagnosed.

"I never take the next step unless they invite me to take the next step, and I always play it positive. Always."

But playing it positive doesn't mean denying someone's fear. "You're so scared sometimes you also need people to just say, 'That's really scary, isn't it?' I mean, the other thing about the cancer thing for me is that sometimes what I really needed was for somebody to be my cheering squad . . . but there were other times when that would be really offensive . . . when it would make me feel isolated. Sometimes what I really needed was people to just hear me."

Susan said, again, it's about asking permission—being open and available to what cancer patients want and need and asking them each time they speak.

"I just have this vision that tomorrow, if everyone in the world started asking for consent, wars would end. The world would change."

Asking permission to share the news that someone has cancer

In the summer of 1995, Ronald Goldberg was creating masks for the *Sesame Street* television show in Minneapolis. He had also just won a grant from the National Endowment for the Arts to hold mask-making workshops in homeless shelters around the San Francisco Bay Area, which is where he grew up and where his parents still lived. He had also started to work as a commercial actor again.

At thirty-one years old, he was living his dream. But in one moment, at a lunchtime audition, his mask was pulled off, revealing a reality worse than any nightmare.

"I was in a big casting room, and I started to feel funny, and a woman was walking toward me, and you know how when a record is played backward? That's what it sounded like, and the

"I did not want to discuss my illness with anyone. It was not that I was in denial, but rather to me, this was just an inconvenience and I figured this too shall pass."

—W.W., prostate cancer survivor

next thing I knew the paramedics were looking down at me and asking, 'Are you all right?' and they rushed me to the hospital, put me in an MRI, and said, 'You have a brain tumor.'"

Ronald flew home to San Francisco where he had the support of family and friends, as well as treatment at one of the world's most respected medical centers, the University of California at San Francisco.

"It was such a shock. It was a week on the couch, and I was floored. I remember talking to people on the phone and hearing only an empty silence on the other end. People were floored that someone they cared about had this, and they didn't know how to respond to it."

His mother responded by learning as much as she could about the disease and offering as much support as possible. His father took a different approach. "I remember my father would talk about it a lot with people, and I did not like that at all. And it was really hard to get through to him."

A private person, Ronald told his father he did not want everyone to know about his illness. He feared people would look at him differently and think, "Oh, there's a dead person."

"Sometimes you'll get questions [from near strangers] like, 'Is everything okay?' and you ask, 'What are you *talking* about?'"

Ronald worried about his father's disclosure of his cancer not just because of the personal implications, but also because of the possible professional and legal ramifications. "If you're going for a job interview, people are going to look at you differently. I mean look at the HIPPA rules [federal laws that prohibit requiring disclosure of individuals' medical conditions], I mean medical privacy is huge."

Ronald said his father continued to tell neighbors and friends at work, even though he asked him not to. "My dad didn't think he was doing anything wrong. It was a huge thing that was going on in his life."

Permission to visit

It was a Friday afternoon when Dana McDaniels got the news that she had breast cancer. (It's uncanny how many people get biopsy results at the start of the weekend, when they have two days to stew and, like a chicken, fall apart before asking all the questions boiling in their minds!)

"I got the phone call from the gynecologist. She told me, 'You have

DCIS and it's invasive.' I asked what that meant, and she said, 'That means it's not so bad—I'll explain it to you at our appointment next week.'"

Dana wanted to know more about the disease before then, so she called a causal friend, a nurse. Dana's eye's widened when she said, "Calling Tina was a big mistake."

Tina demanded, "You have *what*? What did the doctor say, *exactly*?" Tina's dramatic tone scared Dana. "How big is it?" Tina asked. "What treatment did your doctor recommend? Where will you get your second opinion?"

"People who would actually ask if this was a good time to visit helped a lot. I liked it when people would call and make an appointment to come and see me and call an hour before to check that I was up for it."

—S.T., prostate cancer survivor

Even though Tina asked Dana those questions years ago, they stick in her memory like bubble gum under a tabletop. Though intended to help Dana create a plan of action, the questions did anything but help her deliberate.

"I didn't know a thing about breast cancer or tumors." Dana blinked back tears. "I was so shocked when I heard the news that Friday that I don't think I heard half of what the doctor said. And I certainly didn't need the pressure of my friend asking me so many questions; it just made me feel inadequate."

What Dana said she did need was a quiet evening at home with her family—her husband, Steven, and her seventeen-year-old son, Chris. Dana and Steven decided not to tell Chris the news until they knew more about the treatment and prognosis. But they wanted the comfort of his presence, so they rented a movie they knew he would like. Dana wrapped herself in the comfort of her familiar pink bathrobe, soft and soothing, and heaved a sigh of relief.

"I just wanted to relax and sit home with Steven and Chris," she recalled. "When you're told something like that, you just want to find a little safe pocket and stay there for a while."

But she barely had time to start the movie before she heard the doorbell ring.

It was Tina. She was standing there with her husband, Jerome, a doctor. "I just didn't want you to be alone tonight," she said to Dana, who found herself shocked speechless.

Shaken and weakened for the third time that day, but always gentle and polite, Dana invited Tina and her husband to enter her home and have a seat in the spacious but already-darkened living room. Turning on two table lamps, Dana left for the kitchen to make a pot of peppermint tea and compose herself. Chris had disappeared, happy for the excuse to get back on the phone with friends.

"It was great to have meals made, but only if they asked first. I had one well-meaning friend who decided I should go vegan, and what she made was awful. It was great when they put their names on the casserole dishes because it made it easier to return."

—A.M., testicular cancer survivor

Over tea, the two couples did not broach the subject of cancer, but just chattered about news, recipes, mutual friends—the mundane realities that were surreal, not real, to Dana that night.

Tina and Jerome left an hour or so later.

"They didn't make me feel any better. There was no purpose to the visit," Dana said.

It had, however, cleaved her family. Chris was still home, but he was rapt in conversation with his friends. Dana was exhausted anyway and fell into bed, full of dread, partly about how she was going to tell Chris the news about her cancer without scaring him. But she wouldn't have to worry about that for long.

The phone rang first thing the next morning. It was Theresa, the daughter of Tina and Jerome. Chris picked up the phone, groggy with sleep. Though he doesn't remember her exact words, he thinks Theresa said, "I'm so sorry about your mother."

"Theresa's a very emotional person," Chris explained to me, "so she was crying on the phone. She asked if I was okay. I told her I didn't know what she was talking about. Then she was real quiet, and I just said that I had to go."

Chris rushed into his parent's bedroom, but they weren't there, so he ran down the stairs, sprinting toward the kitchen, where he found his father. "What's wrong with Mom?!" Chris demanded.

Steven told him his mother had breast cancer.

"I was really worried," Chris said, "and then I was really confused at the same time because I didn't understand why someone didn't tell me."

Chris felt much better after learning more about the disease and being assured by Steven that his mom would have surgery and be "just fine." But the incident made Dana feel worse than she had when she initially heard the diagnosis. The surprise and intrusion that morning, on top of the shock, anger, violation of privacy, and disappointment from the day before, shook her to her core and rattled the foundation of trust that had supported her family for almost two decades.

"I was worried that Chris would feel that every time something big happened in our family that we weren't sharing everything with him. You know, like we were trying to protect him by leaving him out. Did you kind of feel that way?" she asked Chris, who was looking down at the dining room table where we sat.

"A little bit," he said tentatively.

Dana sighed. "We didn't want to scare you. We wanted to find out more about what was going to happen before we worried you."

Chris continued looking down. "I know," he finally said.

"That was the worst part for me," Dana said apologetically, "because I didn't want you to think that we wouldn't tell you right away."

Chris felt like he had learned a lot from the experience, and he was eager to share his wisdom. His advice to others who hear about a friend's parent having cancer: "Just stay out of it until you know for sure that the family has talked about it. Also, just be there for them. Don't say, 'I know what you're going through,' because obviously you don't. Just be supportive."

As for Dana, she not only lost her innocence that weekend, she also lost a friend.

"Tina called me and apologized, which I'm sure she did after her husband told her what happened with Theresa and Chris," Dana said softly. "I just said, 'Don't worry about it.' I should have been more honest with her about how it affected us, but I wasn't. I'm just too nice."

To this day, Dana cannot face her friend. When she sees her at the supermarket, she turns the other way. She even got caller ID so she could see when Tina was calling. It was so painful for her that she said she has only told two people about the incident, even though it happened years ago.

If Tina had simply called and asked whether Dana and Steven wanted some company that night—and if Tina had asked whether Dana was going to tell Chris—things would have turned out very differently. Dana blamed herself, in part, for not being honest with Tina that night, but most people agree that the onus should be on the friend to ask permission, especially on the day of diagnosis, when patients feel shell-shocked, as if they have been dropped in the middle of a mine field.

Permission to send news

Soon after I myself was diagnosed, my friends started emailing me hopeful articles about new treatments, as well as treatments on the horizon that might help me down the road. I loved my friends for that. They would always read the article first to make sure it did not contain anything that would upset me; if it did, they would excerpt the hopeful parts. They wanted not to scare, but to reassure me.

After I had fully recovered from my treatment, I subscribed to Google news alerts to receive news about lung cancer because there were several drugs, including Iressa, that seemed promising, and I wanted to know more about them, just in case. Mostly, the alerts lifted my spirits. But every once in a while, I would receive an article that mentioned lung cancer's mortality rate, and, depending on my mood, I would be thrown off kilter, sometimes for days or even weeks.

I finally unsubscribed myself and resolved to focus only on success stories. But a few weeks later, someone I used to work with sent me an article written about a woman who had died of lung cancer. It was not what I needed to see. If I had seen the headline on a Google news alert, I would have deleted it immediately.

Before sending articles or news of any kind to a cancer patient or survivor, it's best to ask whether they would like to receive such news. Otherwise, your well-meaning gesture could hurt your friend, and you might never know it.

Permission to share contact information

This seems like it should go without saying, but a real-life example showed me recently that sometimes, acting in haste, people neglect to do what is proper, polite, and even ethical.

Stacey, a friend of mine, told me a story about her twenty-five-year-old cousin, Alex, who had recently been diagnosed with advanced lung cancer.

Alex, who had never smoked a cigarette in his life, had a genetic test to see if he would respond to Iressa, a new drug. He got good news, and immediately he called his mother to share it.

She, in turn, called a friend of hers whose niece, Fanny, had been treated for lung cancer with Iressa. When Fanny found out about Alex, she asked her mother for his email address.

When Fanny emailed Alex, she told him she had experienced awful (and it turns out fairly unusual) side effects from the drug. Instead of instilling hope, the note made him fearful. It also made him angry with his mother's friend for sharing his contact information without asking his permission.

Because no one asked his permission, Alex ended up losing sleep, he said, for several nights. All he wanted at that point was to forget about his cancer—to forget and laugh.

7.
"I need to forget—and laugh!"

Total absence of humor renders life impossible.

—Sidonie Gabrille Colette

WHEN I WAS A NEWS REPORTER, I often heard crude and sometimes cruel jokes lobbed across the open tennis court-size newsroom. Coming from other reporters, editors, or producers, the "funny" stories usually concerned crime victims or disasters. The interesting thing is, I can't recall a single specific example; maybe I purposely put them out of my head once I left the industry. I do remember, however, participating in some of the joking myself. It wasn't so much because I wanted to fit in; it was more so I could cope with the suffering I had to cover on a daily basis.

Though I have forgotten the jokes, I have not been able to erase the sight of a very young Hmong man who drowned himself; his body had been in the Willamette River for five days when they found him, and the smell of decay during the autopsy I observed made me retch outside. I also remember seeing a body bag being carried out of a home after a husband had murdered his wife; I imagined what it was like to be beaten to death, screaming for mercy.

But this is supposed to be happy chapter, isn't it? Indulge me. . . .

Humor is a coping mechanism many people use to deal with tragedy. As Jimmy Buffet sang in "Changes in Latitude," "If we couldn't laugh, we would all go insane."

Hence the gallows humor you hear about among police, emergency room workers, and journalists. Men and women who consistently look into the face of illness, suffering, and death must defuse the fear and anger and insanity they witness.

Though being funny comes more naturally to some than others, most of us have a good enough sense of humor to recognize a good joke. But it can become far more difficult to laugh when you ache, especially when you have cancer and your life is threatened. For one woman, however, cancer actually enhanced her sense of humor—and may have saved her life.

Comedy can cure, this redhead maintains, and according to a study from the Indiana State University of Nursing, humor may enhance the immune system by increasing the body's natural killer cells.

Comedy cures

Saranne Rothberg is no stranger to the gallows humor of a newsroom. She was one of the youngest local television anchorwomen in the nation when CBS targeted her for the fast track to network news. Later she left news for the world of entertainment. As a child she had modeled and acted in both TV commercials and films; now she wanted to work behind the scenes.

"I helped start an independent film company, and I worked in all aspects in development, casting, and internal distribution until it was sold, and then I started my own consulting business," Rothberg explained. "Then I was asked to do the International Children's Summit in New York, and I fell in love with the children. I decided to devote my time to teaching teachers how to teach in a more innovative way, integrating the best of multimedia."

Rothberg's life continued its charmed course. She gave birth to her daughter, Lauriel, created a nonprofit to support the success of teachers, and even received a grant from the government to earn another academic degree.

"Jokes were GREAT! I wanted to laugh. And laugh some more."

—D.R., breast cancer survivor

But then, in 1999, she was diagnosed with cancer. Her daughter was five; she was thirty-four and divorced.

As she wrote in *Coping* magazine, "I fractured my funny bone. I heard 'malignant tumor, surgery, radiation, chemo' and felt as if I'd forgotten how to breathe."

It was a Friday (when else?) when she received her diagnosis, and the doctor said it was too late to assemble his hospital cancer squad. So she found herself with sixty hours to marinate in the bitter terror of cancer. Most people feel more comfortable when actually *doing* something to battle the disease, such as gathering information from doctors or the Internet. But Rothberg had the whole weekend ahead of her, and she had neither a partner nor family nearby to support her. Plus, she had her daughter to care for. What was she to do?

> "One friend became my 'Ministress of Humor.' She sent me funny postcards, called me with off-the-wall jokes, and even brought another friend in to entertain me during an eight-hour chemo session."
>
> —B.D., breast cancer survivor

She came up with not only something to do but, more important, a way to escape. "I had read an excerpt from Norman Cousins's book [*Anatomy of an Illness*]—he was the pioneer of therapeutic humor—when I was in college, and all of a sudden this man's life story flashed before my eyes, and at that moment I said to myself, 'If Norm Cousins can do therapeutic humor then I can do therapeutic humor!'"

She headed straight to the video store and got every standup comedy in stock. "After I put my daughter to bed, for the next twelve hours I laughed and cried through my whole first night, and in that comedy marathon I found my breath in the laughter; I found hope in the laughter.

"I saw that when I was laughing," Rothberg continued, "I felt less fear and less anxiety, and I realized in that distraction that I could use a comic perspective to cope and that I could feel 'normal.' When I watched a comedy, life seemed like I never got a cancer diagnosis; it just seemed fun again."

With her knowledge of Cousins's work and life, and with her very real emotional experience, she started that first new day with a mission. "I asked my daughter if she'd become my humor buddy," Rothberg recalled. "I asked my daughter if she would make an 'appointment' to laugh with me every day no matter what treatments I had to go through, no matter what hospital I was in or what side effects I was having. I wanted to have two times a day where we would put the cancer aside and just laugh."

Rothberg wanted to do that not just for herself but also for Lauriel. Without family nearby or a husband to run interference, Rothberg had to get up every day and parent alone, and she was deeply concerned that cancer not rob Lauriel of her childhood. "I feel a lot of times that children are caught in the cancer crossfire, and as a single parent I was very sensitive to the fact that she have the joy, the wonder, the laughter in her day, and that the weight of the sickness and the fear and the pain of a cancer diagnosis not distort her childhood."

Saranne and Lauriel Rothberg created a daily regimen, a comedy and joy workout not unlike an exercise routine. "The night before when we would go to bed, we would each sit down with the joke book, and we read jokes to ourselves until we found one we liked. Now, you can't read a joke book and not help but laugh and smile—it just puts you in a good mood!

"Laughter was my salve so any funny books, movies, or jokes were so welcome. Anything that reinforced the idea of cancer patients being victims was counterproductive."

—N.D., prostate cancer survivor

"So here we are creating this wellness, smiling to ourselves as we plotted our jokes. Then we would go to sleep without telling each other, which is kind of funny because we share everything and now we're withholding. Then in the morning, whoever woke up first would run into the bedroom of the other person, and before they could say anything, tell them their joke. So your first moments of consciousness were of humor."

Rothberg's voice changed from mischievous to earnest when she said, "What Lauriel and I discovered is that to really appreciate life and not let the little things or the components of cancer get us down, we had to really seek the joy in any given moment, and the comic perspective in any moment. So we developed these highly attuned antenna, like radar, for fun. So the little things in life, like the bullies, like the inability of the chemo nurse to find a good vein—all of those things that happen as a result of growing up in childhood or growing through your cancer journey, they all give you opportunities for comedy or tragedy.

"What we realized," Rothberg considered after pausing, "was that at any minute in our journey, whether it was her personal journey as a child or my cancer, we had the ability to choose joy.

"Now it doesn't mean that you *have to*," she continued, answering my objection before I had time to voice it, "it just means you have the ability to choose."

Rothberg explained that there are plenty of days when she and Lauriel decided to be in a bad mood or cry or feel sorry for their circumstances. "But its not because we're being thrown into it; it's because we decide that's the emotion that will serve us for that time."

"You can lose your hair, your appetite, and forty pounds that will promptly return after chemo. Just don't lose your sense of humor—it's one of your most precious possessions. (My mom taught me that and a valuable lesson it was!)"

—D.K., sarcoma survivor

That sense of choice has allowed both Rothberg and Lauriel to teach others that in the midst of various emotions, they can choose to stop and look for the comic perspective or the lesson. "That is so empowering," said Rothberg, "particularly when you're a child or when you feel like your life is spinning out of control because you have a life-threatening illness."

It was the night that Rothberg sat in the chair at her chemotherapy center and received her first chemical treatment that she came up with the idea to teach others what she and Lauriel had taught themselves. She said she realized she was in that chair for a purpose.

"My first thought was to redefine what it meant to be a patient. You have to take chemo sitting down, but I realized the chair had wheels. I thought, 'Get up, girl, shake your thing!' and so I started to travel, patient to patient, family to family, and ask them if I could give them 'a gift.'"

"Some people were very bitter and they couldn't imagine what kind of gift anyone could give you in a chemo facility. Some people were startled, and some people were so thankful to have a break from the monotony that they were very inviting."

What Rothberg offered patients was the gift of humor. Soon she unwrapped it so thousands of others could enjoy it. From her chemo chair, with a cell phone and laptop computer, she founded the Comedy Cures Foundation. Within a few months, it had grown into a full-service organization, offering a range of programs from a twenty-four-hour joke hotline to laugh-a-grams to live shows featuring New York's hottest comics.

"We guarantee that in our show you will laugh at least a hundred times. And what we do is we have people observe the state of their body, mind, and spirit before, during, and after our show, so you can see in a very real live tangible way the impact these strategies have on you. It's so powerful, it's mind-boggling."

Rothberg said the show works every time, whether viewers suffer acute or chronic disabilities, depression, or debilitating side effects from treatments. "No matter if it's two-year-olds or 102-year-olds, it works every time."

Rothberg described the telephone laugh line as a typical Henny Youngman dial-a-joke; anyone can call to either hear or record a joke.

"What happens across the country is that chemo nurses call it from the chemo ward from the speaker phone so people can hear it. Families call it together. Patients call it at two in the morning when they just can't sleep, when they're so afraid."

Although Rothberg can get people to laugh at her jokes, not everyone has the energy to pick up a phone or can go to one of her shows. (By this time, I couldn't wait to catch the next plane to New York to see Rothberg in action.) So part of the Comedy Cures mission is to help caregivers help their loved ones deliver a belly laugh.

Most of the calls she gets come from friends and family of cancer patients. Their first exasperated complaint is, "We just don't know what to do." Comedy Cures suggests to caregivers that they say to their loved one, "I'd really like to be your humor buddy." The caller is told how to approach the person directly. Rothberg advises caregivers to share with their loved ones how Rothberg, with early stage 4 cancer, decided to make an appointment to laugh with her daughter every day—and to emphasize how much it helped.

Rothberg said sometimes they send out the Comedy Cures button, which says "100 laughs a day—call 1-888-Ha-Ha-Ha-Ha." Or they'll ask callers, "Hey do you know that laughter's really good for you?" and then quote their easy-to-understand synthesis of the studies on the benefits of humor.

Rothberg said research shows that laughing a hundred times is like working out at the gym for ten minutes on a stationary rowing machine or twenty minutes on a stationary bike. She also pointed to several studies that show laughter decreases stress hormones.

"There's a study that shows that for cancer treatment," Rothberg noted, "and when the immune system is under constant stress, it does break down and you become vulnerable to cancer and secondary infections. So it's important to keep your negative stress hormones low and your positive stress hormones high."

Rothberg said scientists have shown that laughing, and even to some degree smiling and thinking humorous thoughts, can positively impact the mind, body, and spirit. "There's a study that shows that your white blood cell count increases; there's an NG4 killer white blood cell that is known to be very effective in fighting cancer, and they've shown that you produce more of those cells when you're laughing."

To experience the benefits of laughter, Rothberg said you have to laugh out loud. That's one of the skills her program teaches. "[Laughing out loud] stimulates your auditory response because you're hearing your own laughter," explained Rothberg. Also, laughter is contagious, "So you're creating health and energy and wellness for other people instead of just hogging it for yourself."

> *"Some friends organized a presurgery girl's night in; we talked and ate and laughed. Everyone brought a dish of frozen food for after-surgery dinners. I didn't need to talk about cancer, although I am sure that would have been all right with them. It was good to be just a woman."*
>
> —T.T., cervical cancer survivor

As if I weren't convinced enough, Rothberg threw in one more study that clinched the sale for me. "If you laugh on the average every day, you will look on the average eight years younger. You never need a face-lift! You're using so many muscles!"

I told Rothberg that if I my cancer comes back, I might not live long enough to need a face-lift. Then I apologized for my gallows humor.

No problem there. "Tumor humor, gallows humor," she almost squealed, "I love it! But I'm very discreet in how I use it because some people aren't ready."

When Rothberg approaches patients in the hospital, she doesn't go in cold and ask, "May I tell you a joke?" She asks if she can give them a gift. She gave me the gift of the following story.

> I was working with a cancer patient, we were in the pre-op room, and she was suited in a gown and shower cap. She looked fearful, anxious, depressed, and a little absurd, and I asked if I could come in and keep her company and if I could give her a gift. I had

some bubbles. The wonderful thing about bubbles is that they take you back to your childhood and also they create breath.

I asked her if she'd blown bubbles before; I told her I use them for stress management. I gave her a bottle and we started to blow bubbles, and I saw she was getting into it, and then we started to have a bubble race. So here we were; it was like the *Lawrence Welk Show,* and we were blowing so hard the bubbles were going out into the hallway, and everyone was curious. Doctors and nurses, they had never encountered bubbles in the hallway before, and the surgeon came in and said, "What's going on?" Then he said, "I have to get some information." I said, "Sorry, not unless you tell her a joke; you're in bubble land: The only way you get information is by telling a joke."

It totally blew his mind. He was in this robotic mood—he'd been performing surgery—and he said, "I can't think of a joke." Well, we told him a joke and he laughed; and then he said, "I just thought of a joke." Twenty minutes later the nurse comes in and said, "Dr. So-and-so, you're getting way behind schedule," and he said, "Don't bother me. Can't you see we're having fun here?"

The three of us walked the patient into the OR together, telling jokes. She got on the table, and she said they told jokes the entire time—the anesthesiologist, the nurses, the doctors. It was like nothing she'd ever experienced. When the surgery was over, the doctor came out to find me in the hospital to tell me she was done. The nurse said, "He never does that, ever!" So when I went to wrap the patient in a blanket, I gave her another present because we always give people presents when they survive their surgeries, and she went home.

The next day I get a phone call from her, to tell me the history of her experience with this doctor. He had never done this: He called her at home that night—he's a New York City doctor—to see how she was feeling, and he told her a joke! And the next time she went in to see him, he had a joke for her, and he said to her, "How's that redhead with the comedy charity? You tell her I said hi if you see her."

She said that totally transformed their doctor-patient relationship.

Rothberg's dream is to transform patients' relationships with their cancer, from one of a sense of imprisonment to a place where you can gain freedom from your pain and fear.

That doesn't mean people with cancer shouldn't experience difficult emotions. "The first thing that we suggest in our program, and again it's from our own experience, is that you can't fix it, you can't rescue them. You can allow space for people to really mourn the loss of the body part or mourn the loss of their hair or mourn the loss of their quality of life, because you can't find the laughter and the joy if you don't let the pain and the anxiety come out."

Rothberg believes the process must be balanced, and she said going through cancer is not all about joy or fear. It must allow time every day for complaining.

Facilitating fun can be as easy as bringing over a pile of movies or as challenging as telling a perfectly timed joke. But there is one thing guaranteed to sink a spirit faster than the speed of light: popping the balloon of hope that keeps the spirit aloft.

8.
"I need to feel hope."

Take hope from the heart of man, and you make him a beast of prey.

—"Ouida" (Marie Louise de la Ramée)

I WAS BORN LORI HOPE CRASILNECK. In 1975, I replaced Crasilneck with Van Kirk when I married a man as romantic as his moniker. We were both working toward philosophy degrees—he as a graduate student, I as an undergraduate. Naïve, idealistic, and madly in love, we knew we would grow old together, watching one another ripen, wither, and wrinkle like young grapes turning to raisins.

After our divorce four years later, I retained only our car, our dog, and his name. Just twenty-five years old and a child of divorce myself, I lost all hope for a love that would last.

But soon I found a career to love, one that enabled me to combine my desire to write and my need to improve the world. After returning to school, I became a television news reporter. Because I had built a name for myself (his), I didn't consider giving it up, even though I felt a faint sense of guilt.

By the time I was thirty-five and had settled into being a single, successful workaholic documentary producer, I decided it was time to take responsibility for my life, give back that which wasn't mine, and move on. I bought a house, got a dog, and dropped Van Kirk, sliding Hope into place as my last name.

Rather than thinking of "Hope" as the soft center in a jawbreaker shell (surrounded by Lori and Van Kirk), *hope* would now define me. And I needed that, badly. Trapped in an enviable full-time job as a staff producer,

I had burned out after making more than fifteen documentaries about social problems such as homelessness, drug addiction, and child sexual abuse. I didn't see how I could survive another project.

Yet hope was suddenly everywhere. When strangers learned my name, they'd often say, "Hope—how nice!" I'd smile proudly, turning my thoughts toward, well, hope. Folks I'd just been introduced to often called me Hope instead of Lori, and I loved it. But once I was diagnosed with cancer, I often feared that there was no longer any hope for Hope.

A hope killer

Back in 1992 when I was making a documentary about right-to-die issues, I considered naming the film *Hoping for a Peaceful End*. Instead, *Help Me Die* won out. I should have added the subhead *A Life-Affirming Look at Death*. Although it may seem like a depressing subject, I found most of the terminally ill people I profiled (most of whom had cancer) inspiring and full of hope. They hoped for a peaceful death. For reconciliation. For pain relief. For the grace to accept care rather than having to provide it. The point is, they hoped.

I hoped I wouldn't get cancer. I halfway expected breast cancer because two of my cousins had had it, so when I was diagnosed with *lung* cancer ten years later, it was a total shock. Even though I had been a smoker in my younger days, it never had occurred to me that I would get cancer almost two decades after kicking the habit. It just didn't seem fair.

"I didn't want to know all the side effects of chemo and Tamoxifen, et cetera. I needed hope and not practical advice."

—S.T., breast cancer survivor

Once diagnosed, I hoped my friends and loved ones would be there for me. I hoped I would survive surgery. I hoped the cancer hadn't spread. And I hoped it wouldn't kill me.

This was a tall order for the kind of cancer I was diagnosed with. My first cousin, Sharon—a beloved woman whom I held in the highest esteem, a down-to-earth woman who was wise, honest, and infinitely kind—had recently been diagnosed with lung cancer. Although hers was more advanced, we had the same form, one that does not respond well to chemotherapy and radiation.

Knowing that, it took great strength for me to muster hope in the face of so much heartbreak and loss. I scoured my soul for any and every thread I could find to weave together a wick for the small candle I needed to light my way. I managed to find strings here and there; I created a mold and eventually summoned the faith to light it.

But some people threatened to extinguish the small flame of hope I had tried to shelter from the winds of ignorance and insensitivity. It wasn't that they were trying to blow out my fire; it was that they were moving so quickly they created a powerful rush of air.

"Lung cancer, ohhhhhhhhhhhhh, that's really bad," some said.

"Are you going to have chemo and radiation?" others asked. I replied matter-of-factly, "No, those treatments don't seem to work well against my kind of cancer because it's so slow growing," all the while fretting to myself that if the surgery didn't work, I'd be outa luck—lights out! I wished people would ask what my treatment was going to be, instead of making assumptions and offering suggestions.

"I wanted to hear success stories. I wanted to hear stories of people who had cancers similar to mine who were now cancer free, had been so for twenty or thirty years, and were living perfectly normal lives."

—B.B., breast cancer survivor

One would expect those who know little about lung cancer to ask such questions about treatment. But I assumed that those who shared my disease would be more sensitive, taking care to instill rather than dash hope. Yet after surgery, when I attended a small discussion group for lung cancer survivors, I met a man who, with one swift breath, snuffed out the fire I had spent months keeping lit.

When I shared my tale, ending with, "My doctor declared me cancer free after my surgery," this man blurted, "Yeah, that's what my doctor told me, and six months later they found another tumor."

His words replayed in my head like the tune "Time to Say Goodbye" during the weeks following my diagnosis. Why had he said that? Perhaps what I had said had hurt him in some way. Maybe he thought I was bragging. But chances are, he was telling the truth to warn me to be vigilant. In this case, though, the truth didn't set me free; it thrust me back into my prison cell of fear.

Fortunately, it was only two weeks later when I met Jill Jordan.

Hope is orange, red, green, and pink

Only about a year posttreatment, I was still raw and frightened when I met Jill Jordan. The loss of my cousin, Sharon, to lung cancer nine months earlier still stung; I missed her, and whenever I thought of her it reminded me that I could meet the same fate. Trying to believe that we would be reunited after death was little comfort (though I must admit that I had some sweet fantasies about seeing her again and talking about the meaning of life over her kitchen table for eternity instead of just a few hours).

"Just because I cried a lot did not mean that I gave up hope."

—R.B., brain tumor survivor

I had learned from talking with Jill on the phone that she had been diagnosed with late-stage lung cancer three years ago, so I expected to find her thin, weak, and pale. During the drive to her home in California's fertile wine country, I steeled myself for a look into the future. I was afraid, but I reminded myself that it was important that I become the mouthpiece for her story.

Walking up the flagstone path to her front door, I noticed flowering bushes on either side that were blooming pink and orange. A hanging plant, also flowering, drew my eyes upward, and I stopped for a moment to take a deep breath before ringing her doorbell. It turned out that wasn't necessary; Jill opened the door before I could ready myself.

Everything about Jill exclaimed "Life!" Her hazel eyes reminded me of moss on a redwood tree. Not thin, but ample, and with a rosy complexion and auburn hair, she radiated warmth.

Inside, a skylight over the kitchen breakfast bar lit a plate of assorted sandwich cookies and a pitcher of iced tea sweating pretty little drops.

"Want to sit outside?" she asked.

Her outside patio was a palate of greens with dollops of cherry, peach, and tangerine. A half dozen hanging geraniums with pink blooms framed a forest green-painted glass-topped table, which reminded me of my kitchen table as a child. An iridescent spiral ornament with a dangling glass bead twirled and caught my eye, as did a mirrored disco ball. Ceramic wind chimes knocked and clucked, and I thought I heard a rooster herald the day, though it was late afternoon.

Everything was bursting with life, but nothing more so than Jill.

"How could someone with stage 4 lung cancer be so happy?" I wondered.

Soon after Jill was diagnosed, her doctor told her that she had just six months to live. "I asked him if I would be around long enough to plan a vacation. He said, 'You can if you want . . .' but the way he said it was like he was programmed for six months, like, 'You can do what you want, but who the heck knows?' But that was the important part to me: 'Who the heck knows?'"

Jill and her husband had saved their money to landscape their backyard, which was wonderfully wild with native plants and tall grasses. "We decided we'd rather go on a family vacation than worry about the yard," she explained, apologizing for a space that, to me, needed no apologies.

"So we rented a house in Hawaii for three weeks," she continued, "a five-bedroom house! We flew our children and our grandchildren over, and we had the most wonderful vacation. In fact, we had the best time of our lives!"

When she returned, Jill underwent another rigorous course of chemotherapy.

"When I was going through chemo, I was on the couch for six months. My exercise consisted of going to the bathroom. My girlfriends would come over. They'd stay all day and make several meals to keep in the fridge. They'd make dinner; we'd chat. They did this pretty often.

"They were so devoted to me; if I wanted to read, that was fine, but sometimes we'd watch a movie together or sit for hours and talk and laugh."

Tears formed in her eyes. "Sometimes they'd take me out for a drive; we'd go to the ocean. They brought me pictures of us together so I could think of them when they weren't there.'"

"Beware how you take away hope from another human being."

—Oliver Wendell Holmes

As much as her friends helped her feel like a beloved human being, the health care system made her feel like a lifeless object.

"You become an invisible entity. Every day is a measurement of a bodily function, checking your blood sugar. I got really sick of numbers. You, the person, have left the building. You become the cancer."

Jill says the chemo was literally killing her, and her doctor said she would have to stay on it the rest of her life. But after six months, she decided that was no way to live. Her doctor had been involved in a study of a new drug, and the study was almost over. He arranged for her to take the then-experimental medication, Iressa.

Almost three years later, Jill's cancer remains in remission.

"We're going to Hawaii again for Thanksgiving," she said. "My goal used to be to turn fifty-nine and to live to see a cure for cancer. My goal now is to be sixty.

"Renewing goals is so important. You prioritize. Even though my doctor says I'm going to die from cancer, doctors don't know everything. When you're born you have a number, and that's up when God says so."

⊇⊇⊇

Six months later, I called Jill, fearful that she would be near death or already gone. But I wanted to know how she was doing. I pushed the buttons on the phone slowly, preparing myself to hear a man's voice.

Instead, I heard a woman who sounded a lot like Jill sing, "Hell-owe-owe!"

"Jill?" I asked.

She was doing wonderfully. Still on Iressa, she was getting a CT scan quarterly to check for new tumors. She had put her house up for sale and was planning to move out of state to Arkansas to be near her niece, who would be her primary caregiver if she were to fall ill again.

She talked of plans to attend a Lion's Club conference at the City of Hope, a health care center in Southern California. I told her how inspiring her sense of hope was to me.

"What else do you have to latch onto?" she asked. "I went back to my oncologist; he's always amazed I'm there. He just has to give me the statistics and the negatives . . . that Iressa can only improve life for three years. But he gave me a wonderful compliment last time. He said I was important in his life because I taught him how to hope, and that has influenced his patients greatly.

"I tell him I can go from one thing to the next; I can hold out and wait until there is a cure."

Jill considers herself realistic; she acknowledges the limitations of Iressa, but she still maintains hope.

"I have a predisposition to look on the brighter side, but when I was faced with the realistic impact of mortality there were two ways I could go. I could either say, 'You're right and I only have this amount of time' and give up control—or latch onto something to give you a glimmer, the spark of hope.

"I'm doing absolutely everything I can to survive. When control is taken away, that's the killer."

Hope heals

"Hope involves being clear-eyed," said oncologist, writer, and journalist Dr. Jerome Groopman. In *The Anatomy of Hope,* a book based on his thirty years as a practicing oncologist and hematologist, Dr. Groopman shares stories of patients who he believes have thrived because of hope—and a few who have failed to thrive because of the lack of it.

In his book, Groopman defines hope as "the elevating feeling we experience when we see—in the mind's eye—a path to a better future. Hope acknowledges the significant obstacles and deep pitfalls along that path. True hope has no room for delusion . . . hope gives us the courage to confront our circumstances and the capacity to surmount them. For all my patients, hope, true hope, has proved as important as any medication I might prescribe or any procedure I might perform."

In Groopman's book, he documents studies that show that "belief and expectation—the key elements of hope—can block pain by releasing the brain's endorphins and encephalin, mimicking the effects of morphine. In some cases, hope can also have important effects on fundamental physiological processes like respiration, circulation, and motor function."

I loved Groopman's book, but just a few days after reading it I learned of a new Australian study that showed for the first time that optimism does not extend the lives of certain cancer patients.

As I have mentioned earlier, I am a philosopher at heart, so I began to analyze the difference between optimism and faith, positive attitude and hope. Few cancer patients want to be told to maintain a positive attitude (see chapter 9, "Telling me to think positively can make me feel worse"), but hope does seem to be essential.

"People were wonderful about talking about the future in a natural way. It was helpful because I could see that they were assuming I would be around in the future."

—D.S., lung cancer survivor

It seems that a "positive attitude" pertains more to getting well, being cured, or surviving, while "hope" can apply to a myriad of conditions. We can hope for comfort rather than pain, for example, even if we don't believe our cancer will be cured.

"While there's life, there's hope."

—Proverb

In any event, I wanted to hear what Dr. Groopman had to say about hope and, more important, the dearth of hope. I asked him via telephone what he believes are the most common hope killers.

"One is the view of illness as punishment, you know, 'This is happening to me because I did something wrong,' and in a religious framework that can happen because of a distorted theology. And in a nonreligious framework, unfortunately, there's an enormous amount of misinformation about the mind-body connection." Groopman said that there is a whole literature in the field of cancer that maintains that people get the disease because they focus their anger, depression, or resentment in their body, and that if they can only let it go and find love, their tumor will spontaneously remit.

"That's completely fallacious; it's wrong, it has no scientific basis, and it's very, very cruel to the patient," said Groopman, "because you're basically saying you're responsible for your cancer and because you're having negative thoughts or because you're despairing, you're going to be responsible for your own demise."

Dr. Groopman said the Australian study was flawed for several reasons. (In my mind, one of the reasons was that it studied individuals with lung cancer, one of the most wicked and, until recently, more treatment-resistant cancers.) Dr. Groopman said that with only 179 patients, the study was too small to be considered statistically valid. Also, it studied optimism rather than hope.

"Optimism is very different from hope. An optimist says everything's going to turn out just fine. Hope is very different, it sees all the problems and all the issues you're facing and then it chooses what appears to be the best path based on information."

A lack of hope may impair health as much as an abundance of it bolsters health. In "An Essay on Hope" from *Fire, Your Will to Live* by Ernest and Isadora Rosenbaum, the authors cite a phenomenon called "self-willed death or bone pointing," which is practiced in (ironically) Australia, among Aborigines, as well as in other South Pacific cultures.

"In such cases, a tribal witch doctor casts a spell similar to that observed in voodoo . . . causing the victim to suffer paralyzing fear, withdraw from society, and die within a short time. Of course the witch doctor can only be effective if the potential victim believes in the power of the curse."

In the same way, say the Rosenbaums, a person with an illness can be adversely affected when doctors and nurses project a sense of hopelessness, or when family and friends cannot hide their fears.

Maintaining hope may come more easily to those who have cancer themselves than to their caregivers. But it's essential that caregivers keep hope alive—if not hope for survival, then at least hope for a peaceful end.

False hope

When my cousin Billee was dying, one of her friends said he feared she was holding onto "false hope"—that she was in denial because she was leaving her son. I didn't see any harm in holding out hope until the very end, but her friend worried that she wouldn't have time to come to terms with the fact that she was dying. I knew Billee, and I knew she had come to terms with death and had made all the preparations. I felt upset with her friend. And I wondered, "What is false hope, anyway?"

"There's no such thing as false hope," said psychologist Lawrence LeShan, the conviction in his voice raising his volume a few decibels. "Hope bears its own validity. False hope is a meaningless hope and a disruptive one.

"Hope is only the love of life."
—Henri-Frédéric Amiel

"What is false hope?" continued the author of *Cancer as a Turning Point,* who has seen dozens of "terminally ill" cancer patients die not of cancer but of some other malady. "It means the person is not going to get better, which means the other person has a crystal ball and knows more about the subject than God. So anybody who says you have false hope is an arrogant son of a bitch. You can quote me on that."

Therapist Halina Irving, who survived the Holocaust and the death of her mother, sister, father, and son, has never given up hope. She believes that, regardless of what doctors say, people always find something to hope for, like feeling at peace, a better world, or a death without pain. How can hope be false, when it is as much a part of the human experience as birth or death?

"People hope naturally," said Irving. "You don't have to tell them to hope. When you work with dying people, it's painful in a way to see how hard it is to kill hope; they've been given a terminal prognosis—they've been told they're going to die, they are dying, hospice is on the scene, there is no more treatment. And they'll say, 'I know, I know," they'll acknowledge it, but ten minutes later they'll say, 'Did the doctor call? Did the doctor look at the last X-rays?' That's hope."

Hope helps people who have had cancer—or people who haven't—live a more fulfilling life. But it is feeling normal, without having to hide our doubts or put up charades, that makes us feel like we really belong in the land of the living.

9.

"Telling me to think positively can make me feel worse."

*I was going to buy a copy of The Power of Positive Thinking,
and then I thought: What the hell good would that do?*

—Ronnie Shakes

WHEN NATALIE BORNE OPENED her front door and saw me standing in my faded blue cotton UCLA warm-ups, her eyes lit up as if I were Publishers Clearinghouse come to grant her $10 million. Her waist-high Labrador retriever, Ebony, almost knocked me over with his exuberance. Natalie had to tell him quite firmly to sit so she and I could take a good look at one another. We had been trying to get together for weeks, and we were excited to finally meet.

I had sent out an email, which Mimi Roth at the Ida and Joseph Friend Cancer Center had distributed; someone on Mimi's list had forwarded it to Natalie. The message asked cancer survivors to email me stories about words and actions that helped or hurt.

Natalie's first message to me read: "I would be willing to share my experience of the last year. Briefly, I have had two unrelated types of cancer this year, over fifty visits to doctors, every range of side effects, and the best friends and support in the world."

I called her, expecting to hear complaints, which was, after all, part of what I was seeking. (As Lily Tomlin said in Jane Wagner's play, *The*

Search for Signs of Intelligent Life in the Universe, "I personally think we developed language because of our deep inner need to complain.") But once I heard what Natalie had been through, I wasn't sure I would be able to listen to her entire story when we met.

Ultimately her bright blue eyes, joyous smile, and unflappably positive attitude made her suffering almost easy for me to bear, especially since, by the time we met, she was back to full mental and physical health.

"To tell me, someone with cancer, 'you're going to be fine' meant nothing to me. I don't know if I'm going to be fine, and no amount of positive thinking is going to change that. I don't consider myself a pessimist, that's just the reality of the situation."

—N.N., prostate cancer survivor

Welcoming me into her khaki Craftsman home, she led me straight into the kitchen, seating me at a glass table (through which we could keep an eye on Ebony). "Tea?" she asked, and while she brewed some up, she served me a piece of her life.

Natalie had been diagnosed with melanoma fourteen years earlier after finding a suspicious-looking mole on her left thigh. Doctors removed the lesion from her shapely thirty-two-year-old leg, and she went about her business. Divorced with two children, she soon returned to work. With her energy back, she resumed her athletic routine of bicycling, jogging, and weight training. Cancer had been just a blip on the radar.

But thirteen years later, several more blips appeared, presaging what felt like imminent disaster. The first torpedo hit when she was laid off during the dot-com bust. Then her lawn mower mangled a digit on her right hand.

"When I lost half my finger, I almost gave Ebony away because she was distracting me and I felt like, 'I can't do this; I lost my job and now the dog . . .' But then I called the people I was going to give her to and said, 'I can't do it; I love this dog too much.'"

Soon after, Natalie found a second mole on her back; again, melanoma. The treatment: interferon—twenty strong doses in a row.

"The worst thing wasn't nausea; it was that my bones hurt," she winced. "There were days I couldn't even get out of bed." But most days she made herself get up, with Ebony's help.

"I had to get up every morning to take him for a walk. Just knowing there's someone or something else depending on you sort of gets you out of your fog. Just his devotion to me . . . I love him for that."

Her two sons were devoted, too, taking her to doctor's appointments and cooking and cleaning for her. But it was wearing on them.

"My sons are under so much pressure after this ordeal. Do you know how much my son who lives in town would have appreciated someone taking the load off his hands, someone coming over doing the cooking or staying up with me at night when I was in pain?"

Natalie was supposed to stay on interferon for a year, but after a month she cut down to half the dose and soon stopped the treatment completely.

"What, I'm going to give up a year to gain a year of life?" she asked.

"Some days are lousy, and I can't imagine having to spend those days trying to psych myself out with positive psychobabble. That would take far too much energy, and I can't imagine the pressure if I believed a negative thought could cause my cancer to come back."

—R.K., leukemia survivor

Just when she felt things couldn't get much worse, doctors found a lump in her breast. This was too much. She told them she would come back in three months.

She decided to take a vacation, and she headed to Telluride for its famed film festival. There she met a man from New York named Michael, whose company she enjoyed and whom she wanted to see again.

"When I came back home, I called him and said, 'I really need to know how to process this because I really thought you were a wonderful person, and it's okay if it's nothing more, but I need to know.' And he said, 'You're one of the sweetest and most refreshing people I ever met, but I can't date you.'"

"Why not?" Natalie asked. It was because she was of a different faith. So she asked him to introduce her to three books about his religion so she could become educated about it.

Soon after, Michael took her on a trip to Barcelona. But at the end of the trip, he still felt strongly that he wanted to be with a woman who shared his faith.

Natalie came home disillusioned and devastated. On top of her heartbreak, she had cancer to cope with. "Right before I went on the trip, I'd gotten the results that it was in my lymph nodes, so I came home, and the first thing the doctor said to me is, 'You need to make peace with those you have bad feelings about.' He said that the people who live are the ones who make peace with their past."

Having been directed to think positively, she reached out to Michael, in spite of her pain, fear, and anger. The two became friends, talking on the phone and corresponding.

"I resented most of the things about positive attitudes and cheering up and making an effort. I did try to be reasonable because I had two sons, twelve and fourteen, but I didn't feel it was someone's place to tell me how to react, if they hadn't been in my shoes."

—S.T., kidney cancer survivor

"He was very sweet and he would listen to me, and I guess I wanted something more at that time because I loved him so much," said Natalie. "I knew we weren't going to work out as a couple, but his emails meant so much to me, and I told him how much they meant."

Natalie had fallen in love not only with Michael but also with his religion, Judaism. She had started going to study groups, which she said helped her healing and inspired her deeply. "It's the most wonderful journey I've taken. It's the best thing that's happened to me," she smiled.

About eight months into her friendship with Michael, Natalie told him, 'You know, I finally came to the realization that you were brought into my life to lead me to this path.'"

Soon after, he broke off their friendship again.

Natalie believes that she and Michael were not meant to be together, but that truly, his purpose was to introduce her to his religion. That was important, she says, because she was going to get ill yet again and was going to need more spiritual support than ever. A lumpectomy had failed to remove all the cancer in her breast, so she had to undergo another surgery.

She also opted for chemotherapy and radiation. She tried to keep up a good front—her perennially positive attitude.

"Then I started losing my hair," she recalled. "Two months after the chemo, people would call and ask, 'How are you doing?' and you don't want to say, 'Fine,' because you're not, yet you don't want to keep complaining. So I always tried to have something positive to say. But it got to the point where I really didn't want to act anymore."

Natalie was fortunate to have a best friend who completely accepted her, in sickness and in health. "From day one I knew that she wouldn't judge me no matter what I said. She knew the old me, and she knew this was a phase I was going through and that I really needed support, so it really felt good that out of all my friends I knew I had one friend I could just unload on."

Natalie said her friend called every day, even though she lived a busy life twenty-five hundred miles away. "She just absorbed it every day and felt the pain with me. I had only known her three or four years, but our friendship solidified because of that. She doesn't think she did anything to help me get better, but she did.

"She's the only one who each day would reach out to me, I didn't have to reach out first. She'd ask, 'How are you doing today? How do you feel? What are the meds doing?' And she would tell me, 'You're amazing! You're so strong! I know you can do this!'

"She made me feel like I wasn't posing. I could say negative things—be negative—and she wouldn't judge me."

Natalie said her friend's support got her through the toughest time of her life. Now that it's over, she has resolved to change her life and start her own business.

"It's airbrush tanning," she explained. "It's a sugar-based solution that can be airbrushed on, and it lasts for five to seven days. I'm going to promote health—my primary goal is to show people they can have a healthy look without going out to the sun."

Natalie was giddy about the prospect of leaving her high-pressure job in the technology industry for a vocation that could help prevent more cases of melanoma. She invited me to come back for a free tan once she got her tanning studio set up. She wanted to test it out on a few friends so she could develop her skills before setting up shop.

We stayed around her kitchen table for another hour, talking about life-threatening illnesses with an insider's perspective, then we gave one another a big, warm good-bye hug at her door. Ebony licked my hand. Six months later, I got an email from Natalie inviting me over for an airbrush tan.

When being negative can be positive

You would think one would feel uncomfortable standing naked in front of a near stranger, but I was relaxed as I stood in my birthday suit getting misted by a dye that would make me look like I'd spent a week in Cabo San Lucas. Cancer is a strong binder; it seems to melt differences as it fuses people together.

After my "tanning," I felt comfortable enough with Natalie to confide that I was nervous because I had just received word that a recent pap smear showed abnormalities. I would have to undergo another procedure to further diagnose my condition, which was likely precancerous.

"Well, you just have to have a positive attitude!" she said cheerfully.

"You know, Natalie," I said as kindly as I could, "there's some question about the value of positive thinking." I was thinking of the study Australian researchers had just published, which showed that lung cancer patients who maintained a positive attitude lived no longer than those who didn't.

After I told her about the study, she said defensively, "But my doctor told me I had to think positively. That's why I followed up with Michael after he broke my heart, because my doctor said I needed to be positive and not carry that anger around with me."

I felt awful because I realized I may have shattered her faith. "I am so sorry," I said. "Thinking positively can be a wonderful thing, but a lot of people with cancer don't like to be told to think positively because it can be so hard when you have a legitimate reason to feel horrible. And when people can't think positively, sometimes they feel like they've failed and that they're making their cancer worse."

Dr. Jimmie Holland has seen that happen far too often. The former chair of the Department of Psychiatry and Behavioral Sciences at Memorial Sloan-Kettering Hospital in New York, she founded the field of psycho-oncology, which looks at the side of cancer that tries to eat away our hearts and minds, not just our bodies. She wrote in her classic *The Human Side of Cancer* about the "Tyranny of Positive Thinking."

"For most patients, cancer is the most difficult and frightening experience they have ever encountered. All this hype claiming that if you don't have a positive attitude and that if you get depressed you are making your tumor grow faster invalidates people's natural and understandable reactions to a threat to their lives.

"This problem has been brought to me by well-meaning families who say, for example, 'You have to help Dad. He's going to die because he isn't positive and he's not trying.' On meeting Dad, I see that he clearly is a stoic, a man who copes well in his own quiet way. Maintaining a positive attitude just isn't his style. Insisting that he put on a happy face and cope in a way that would be foreign to him would actually be an added burden. To rob him of a coping mechanism that has worked before seems unfair, even cruel."

Indeed, one psychology professor at Wellesley College wrote a book maintaining that thinking negatively can be a plus for some people. In *The Positive Power of Negative Thinking,* Julie K. Norem, PhD, details her scientific research on "defensive pessimism" and tells stories of "people who have harnessed the power of their negative thinking to increase their self-esteem and make significant progress toward their personal goals."

"I am not a power-of-positive-thinking person. I am a complex human being with intricately woven responses to optimism, pessimism, hope, fear, faith, and God. I detest when people tell me that I have to think optimistically."

—D.B., breast cancer survivor

Dr. Holland says telling a patient to think positively can actually hurt.

I interviewed her when she came to San Francisco for a colleague's retirement tribute.

"I think this issue of being positive suggests a kind of Pollyanna state that you should keep all the time," she explained. "But we want people to say when they're depressed and don't feel good—or else we're not going to be able to help them."

Dr. Holland said it's completely normal to feel depressed and think negatively, cancer or no cancer. "You just feel down sometimes. Nobody has the same mood all the time—you have down days, I have down days."

Therapist Halina Irving offered a historical perspective. "Over the centuries human beings have dealt with their fear of catastrophe or disease by saying to themselves, 'This happened to that person because they thought negatively or they led a stressful life.' In past centuries, they said it was because they had unclean thoughts, because they were immoral, because they were witches, because they were bad people.

"I believe that the connotation of 'badness' is attached to so-called negative thinking," continued Irving, "and if you're a good person, then you'll think positively, and if you think positively, then you have a better chance of getting well. It's blaming the victim."

Irving says we blame the victim—the person who is sick—because it makes us feel safer. If we assure ourselves that keeping stress at bay will keep cancer away, we feel like we have some control over our fate. But this does a great disservice to the patient, says Irving, because now, "not only do they have to suffer the pain of the cancer, the fear that they're going to die, and the pain of treatment, but also the reality that they will be seen by others in a negative light if they don't get better."

Understanding this, I still felt badly about sharing with Natalie what I had learned about the tyranny of positive thinking. I had burst her bubble, telling her, in effect, that she should not have acted upon her doctor's advice, which had resulted in her getting hurt again by Michael.

"I am so sorry, Natalie," I apologized. "But you know, there's another book out, and I interviewed the author, that talks about the importance and value of having hope, as opposed to thinking positively."

I explained that we can have hope even while maintaining a negative— or sometimes simply realistic—attitude. For instance, if you're dying of cancer, you can still hope for pain relief. If you have a difficult-to-treat cancer, you can still hope for new treatments.

"Oh, my God, that's great!" she cried, eyes widening and lighting up like the first day I met her. "It has been so hard for me to think positively all the time, and having hope makes so much more sense! Thank you for telling me about that!"

I finally released my breath, returning her brilliant smile. She added, "And I hope your tests turn out okay. You don't need to think positively, but I'm hoping for you!"

I left Natalie's house that day feeling more hopeful than ever. She remained upbeat and cheerful throughout, finding something positive about everything we'd discussed. But we both realized that feeling accepted—being able to think negatively with impunity—had enabled us to better accept whatever would come our way. And it would make us feel more confident about whatever future decisions we would have to make about our health.

10.

"I want you to trust my judgment and my treatment decisions."

Advice is the only commodity on the market where the supply always exceeds the demand.

—Author unknown

WHEN MY FRIEND MARILYN flashes her gorgeous and disarming half-moon smile, her mouth stretches across her entire face (I guess that's where the expression "ear-to-ear grin" comes from). But it's not just her mouth that radiates like an unearthly orb; her eyes are pure neon.

I fell in love with Marilyn's face and her generosity of spirit when we waited on tables in the late '70s at Culpepper's, a chic bistro in St. Louis's Central West End. The floor-to-ceiling windows invited all within to see and be seen; the small spotlights over each table and the chrome and mirrors throughout added flash and glamour.

I had just gotten my BA in philosophy, had married my college sweetheart, and was considering grad school so I could teach at the university level. With a master's degree in special education, Marilyn had just put her short teaching career on hold.

We had way too much fun in those days—dancing, partying (as they now call it), doing all those things young people do when they are living for the moment. Marilyn and I shared an intense joie de vivre, and we forged an instant friendship.

One night soon after we met, she took me to Balaban's, the most exclusive restaurant in the neighborhood and treated me to lobster. She'd gotten a fifty-dollar tip, which was not terribly unusual for Marilyn; her smile made people want to throw money at her.

Her energy level was as high as her smile was wide. And when I needed her energy, it was there for me.

That spring, my husband and I decided to separate; we had married too early. The Saturday morning I was to move out came too soon, also; numb and indecisive, I was unable to move.

"I had a long talk with a friend who is a homeopathic practitioner. He kept encouraging me to deny chemo, that it was poison. It didn't help me at all. My choice wasn't respected, and I was left with a sinking suspicion that I may be choosing to poison myself."

—T.A., stomach cancer survivor

Marilyn showed up, scrambled three extra large eggs in a cast iron skillet, buttered some white toast, and said, "Eat this." Then she started her signature whirl; like a dervish, she picked up shoes, vases, photos, makeup, and notebooks, asking "Keep? Throw away?" Quickly but deftly, she wrapped them in newspaper and packed them away or placed them in a box for Goodwill.

Marilyn was there for me in a way no one else had been. She judged neither me nor my decision; she accepted what was happening and simply stayed beside me. I felt like I owed her my life.

So twenty-five years later, when she called me and told me her mother was dying of breast cancer and asked for my help, I eagerly agreed. I would have jumped on a plane and flown the three thousand miles to New Jersey had she asked. But that's not what she wanted. Knowing I had recently lost a dear friend to colon cancer and a beloved cousin to breast cancer, she thought I would understand what she was going through.

I did, sort of. I volunteered what I thought would help. I listened and tried not to offer any advice, attempting to give her my full attention and share her pain. I think I mostly succeeded. But in one way, I may have failed (though she assures me now I did not, the sweet person that she is). Not having had cancer myself at that time, I don't think I understood what her mother needed.

What I did wrong was to push my beliefs onto her mother, a woman who was clearly dying. Rather than accept what was happening to her, I challenged it, thinking perhaps I could control it and spare Marilyn the loss of her mother, a loss I had recently experienced.

I asked, "Have you ever heard of IP-6? It's a formulation made of the same substance in brown rice. It's supposed to have tumor-fighting properties."

I don't recall when I first read about IP-6, but I think I discovered it in some of the research I did for my dear friend Missy. Though not a scientist, I did work as a medical journalist for a number of years and considered myself skilled at critical thinking. After reading the literature about IP-6, I thought it might actually shrink tumors.

But it was expensive. Even so, I bought a large bottle and overnighted it to Marilyn, who was staying with her mother. I included a note advising that her mother should take sixteen capsules a day (a normal dosage is four), that it might do some good.

I regret doing so. Probably the last thing her dying mother wanted to do was swallow sixteen more pills each day when she was undoubtedly already swallowing many to treat her pain. And she certainly had made her treatment decisions long ago.

When Marilyn's mother died a few weeks later, I received the half-empty $100 bottle of IP-6 back.

ㄹㄹㄹ

Did I get the message back then? Well, I had not yet had cancer. Several years later, when my cousin Sharon was diagnosed with lung cancer, I sent her some IP-6, too. Although this time I sent it soon after Sharon's diagnosis, and I sent a powder that could be dissolved in water, I still had no right to push upon her my idea of what I thought would work. "I want to send you this," I said. And because she was so kind and generous, Sharon said, "Okay." She placated me because she knew I needed to do something for her.

I didn't understand this at all until I had cancer myself and people started asking me whether I had heard about this or that mushroom. My husband, David, who may have been as anxious as I before surgery, went to the vitamin shop to pick up some IP-6 for me. The owner of the store started pleading with David not to let me have surgery until I had tried a new something-or-other, shark's gonads or something.

David rushed home, eager to share the news, but I did not want to hear it. I believed in IP-6, and I wanted the blasted tumor out of my body as soon as possible. I was not willing to gamble my life on something unproven.

That was when I finally understood that once someone makes a treatment decision, more advice only confuses or scares them; it can also undermine their confidence in their doctors or advisors. When I had cancer, I needed to trust those who held my life in their hands.

I felt ashamed and angry with myself for doing what I had done to Marilyn and also to Sharon, who seemed to go to her grave with only love toward me. When I heard stories like Margaret Stauffer's, I felt even worse. But hearing that she was able to forgive those who hurt her helped me forgive myself.

How are we to know what to do if no one tells us?

Just ask me

Margaret Stauffer came to the Wellness Community not as a cancer patient, as most do, but as a professional. With a background in mental health as a marriage and family therapist, she started working first with diabetics. "But, having had a lot of cancer in my family, I came to read Gilda Radner's book, where I learned about the Wellness Community. I found there was a position available in San Diego, and so I started there in 1992."

When Stauffer moved to the Bay Area three years ago, she transferred to the Wellness Community in Walnut Creek because, as she said, "I can't imagine working anyplace else."

As the program director of the nonprofit agency, she develops all the educational program calendars and stress-reduction programs, supervises the clinical teams, facilitates some of the support groups, and reaches out to the community to make people aware of the services the Wellness Community offers.

I drove to the suburb of Walnut Creek to interview Stauffer to gather information for this book and to sit in on one of the Wellness Community's support groups. I expected to hear Stauffer tell stories from her decade of experience working with cancer patients, but instead, I heard what I would hear from almost every authority I consulted for this book: a personal story from her own life that helped her truly understand and feel compassion for others.

Stauffer told me the story of her mother, a sweet and kind woman who had endured the rigors of breast cancer three times, but who never talked with her daughter about her fears or her poor prognosis. She did talk with Stauffer about other emotions, however.

"When my mother was dealing with her third recurrence of breast cancer, I remember a lot of well-meaning friends bringing her different books about what she should do to recover from cancer. And I think she always had the feeling that people thought if she would just do all the things they suggested that she would be okay.

"Some friends recommended herbal remedies, which could be very dangerous when mixed with regular medications. Others gave me books to read about cancer. The only one that I enjoyed was The Red Devil. *It was written by a cancer patient who survived three bouts of breast cancer."*

—S.W., breast cancer survivor

"It was almost a way of blaming the person with cancer for being in the state that they were in," continued Stauffer, obviously pained. "And even though my mother was a very gentle, quiet person, she finally was pushed to the point where she told people she didn't want anything that was self-help related—that she had made her decision about what she was going to do, and it was not helpful for her to get all these suggestions."

I asked Stauffer what that was like for her mother.

"She felt really awful about being encouraged to try so many things when she was barely hanging on to being able to do what she thought was appropriate as far as medical treatment, and managing her stress and dealing with the emotions of having a third recurrence."

Stauffer said her mother had no intention of trying what her friends suggested—such as adopting restrictive and severe diets or particular ways of thinking. Stauffer said her mother had her own ideas.

"What kind of ideas?" I asked.

"I think that for her, the most important thing was being able to have music, to express herself through that. She was a pianist. And to enjoy the beauty that she saw around her and her home. She found animals very comforting."

I asked whether her mother had given up hope of surviving. "Oh, no," she insisted, "but she was tired of people telling her how to do what. I think that was the peeve. There's a difference between saying, 'This was really helpful for me, do you want to hear about it?' and, 'This is what you *should* do; I've known people who have been cured of cancer by doing this.' You know, that sort of desperate search."

I agreed and added, "It's a desperate attempt by the friend or loved one, in part because they're so scared and they feel powerless. And they want control."

"Very much," agreed Stauffer.

"But it's not the time to take control from somebody," I concluded.

"Not helpful: 'Maybe you should stop drinking diet pop and try these special vitamins that worked for my cousin Irving's prostate.'"

—B.C., breast cancer survivor

Again, it had come back to asking permission. Stauffer said, "I think it's more than courtesy—asking permission to learn if the person wants to hear it or not. Because some people are very interested in finding out about all the alternatives; they want to try all of them and that's wonderful. But it's finding out what the person wants—what's helpful to them."

I left the Wellness Community that afternoon feeling guilty about having pushed my beliefs onto people who had been so vulnerable, so needy. But my intentions were pure, and I had acted out of love. And I felt better as I realized that I was alive, here and now, and had been given an opportunity to give a voice to those who should never be pushed to the point of saying, "I don't want to hear about it."

Giving cancer patients the opportunity to say yes or no to suggestions about treatment is another way you can help them live happier and possibly longer lives.

11.

"I want compassion, not pity; comfort, not advice."

If you want others to be happy, practice compassion.
If you want to be happy, practice compassion.

—The Dalai Lama

I DON'T REMEMBER HOW OLD I was when I first discovered what made me feel completely different from everyone else. But I do remember feeling freakish, hideous, and branded because of two small birthmarks. Fortunately, I was able to hide them beneath my clothing, and I eventually had them removed surgically. But the shame had taken root and had remained buried so deeply that I never trusted anyone with my secret. My mother took the secret to her grave, and I do not think my father ever knew how ashamed I was. It seemed so silly, after all.

But if I realize now how silly it was, why haven't I told anyone?

Humans are the most social of animals. In our earliest day as *Australopithecus,* if we didn't fit into the group and were banished, we would die. We carry that with us today. "No man is an island," said John Donne, and although Simon and Garfunkle countered with, "I am a rock, I am an island," we all know what these expressions mean.

We do not want to be alone (that is not to say we do not enjoy solitude, but that is a different conversation altogether), and we do not want to *feel* alone. My birthmarks—small supernumerary nipples that would have been covered by my breasts if they had grown large enough—made me feel completely different from everyone else. I feared I would be laughed at and ostracized if anyone knew. I felt cursed, and I carried the burden alone all through my childhood and adolescence until a surgeon replaced the birthmarks with two little scars when I was eighteen.

"Try to understand that people with cancer need compassion, not pity. We need constructive interactions, not token activities and words. Kindness, a simple quality, can go a long way. Patience IS a virtue when being with cancer patients. A friendly hand to hold works miracles."

—J.K., breast cancer survivor

Even after having the birthmarks removed, I flushed with shame when hearing the joke, "Martinis are like a woman's breasts: one's not enough and three's too many." I had a secret that made me different.

Thirty years later, being diagnosed with lung cancer was the closest I had come since then to experiencing such isolation, fear, and shame. I had smoked in my youth, and although my oldest friends knew that, most who had known me for less than two decades had no idea. Over and over, when I shared my diagnosis, unwitting colleagues and acquaintances would gasp, "But you never smoked!" Over and over, I would admit, sheepishly, "Well, yes I did, but I quit almost twenty years ago."

Sometimes I would sense they were judging me. "Only idiots smoke," I would imagine them thinking, and I would then think myself an idiot. My spirit would shrink. Other times, I would just feel different. But when people said, "I used to smoke, too," I would feel a sameness, a sense of compassion, like they knew that they could wind up in the same boat.

That's partly why I felt so comfortable when I interviewed Jill Jordan, a lung cancer survivor. She said she hated it when people asked her how long she had smoked.

As psychiatrist Jimmie Holland points out in *The Human Side of Cancer,* "It makes no sense to blame the person who is ill. Being ill makes one feel alone enough, and being blamed adds to a feeling of distance and isolation, of somehow being 'different' from others in a way we've never experienced before."

We all need to feel a sense of equivalence and camaraderie.

And compassion.

Compassion defined

Pema Chödrön wrote, "Compassion is not a relationship between the healer and the wounded. It's a relationship between equals . . . [it] becomes real when we recognize our shared humanity."

The "com" in *compassion* is a prefix used to mean "with or together," as in combine or compact. Combined with "passion," *compassion* means to "feel" or "suffer" with.

Although compassion is often defined as or used as a synonym for "pity" in dictionaries, I see a big difference. Who wants to be pitied, after all? The implications are very different. I met a man of great compassion who explained it beautifully.

Compassion and pity

It was 6:30 A.M. and still dark in the high-ceilinged industrial kitchen of the Santa Sabina Retreat Center. Just outside San Rafael, California, on the campus of Dominican University, Santa Sabina had promised the peace, quiet, and comfort writers yearn for.

Groggy, I turned the corner from the large stainless steel table in the middle of the darkened kitchen and shuffled into the long narrow pantry, where four refrigerators and freezers buzzed. My heart jumped; in my pre-caffeinated state, the stately man in a dark green flannel robe just inches away might have been a bear. He immediately assuaged my fear with his happy black eyes and joyful, almost silly grin.

"Good morning!" he whispered loudly. "Good morning," I replied. "Beautiful morning!"

Though we were different genders and he towered at least a foot above me, and though we likely hailed from different universes, I felt a kinship with him immediately. It wasn't until after two or three minutes of small talk that I learned he was an esteemed priest who had traveled across the country from North Carolina to lead the Easter Retreat, which was to start later that day.

I told him I was a writer and that I was there working on a book about what to say and do to help people with cancer, and he nodded knowingly as he listened. We chatted for a few minutes about well-meaning friends and family who sometimes inadvertently and unintentionally make their loved ones feel worse, and I knew that, even though he had never suffered from cancer himself, he understood what it was like to need compassion.

As we were about to leave the kitchen with coffee cups in hand, we realized we had not even exchanged names. "I'm Jude Siciliano," he said, shaking my left hand with his own.

The next day I awakened with an urge to ask Father Siciliano about the difference between compassion and pity. I was about to look for him, first in the square interior courtyard garden, blooming red, white, and pink, then among the long oak tables in the dining room—when he appeared in the hallway just outside the kitchen.

"I know this is pretty random," I began, "but I've been thinking for days about the difference between pity and compassion, and for some reason I think you have something to say about that."

"I do," he said, eyes smiling. We walked through the glass doors to the grassy rear courtyard and sat at a picnic table covered by a wide canvas umbrella. I turned on my tape recorder, and as he spoke, I watched this warm man in sweats and slippers transform instantly into a scholar.

"My friend had an answer for everything, and her concern was that I was getting the 'right' medical treatment. I know she loved me and wanted to help, but I felt she was undermining my intelligence and treatment program. I avoided her and her 'superiority of knowledge.' Her actions added to my depression."

—H.D., colon cancer survivor

"When I do reflections with people in scripture groups and people have a chance to reflect on their reactions," he began, "one of the words they take offense at is the word 'pity'—like 'Jesus having pity'—and it's used a lot in the New Testament. But its an Old Testament term, too," he added quickly.

"So in the New Testament, Jesus has pity on people who are diseased or in need, as in 'Jesus had pity on him and he reached out and touched the man and the man could see.' But people in groups say, 'I don't like the word pity because it sounds condescending, and who wants pity?'

"Pity is what you do when you toss some money to someone in the street," Father Siciliano continued. "Somehow there's this feeling of aboveness."

A better translation of the word that is used in the Bible is "compassion." Father Siciliano explained: "The Greek word is *compassion,* and it means a feeling that comes from the womb or the bowels. It's what a parent feels when a child falls and cries—that instinctual feeling that arises for something you want to respond to. A woman once told me when her child falls and she hears it crying, the milk in her breast flows. That's physical *and* emotional."

He went on to talk about the Latin origin of *compassion,* which means to suffer with. He explained that it avoids the sense of looking down on someone, as if you're above them. Compassion, he said, is about sharing the pain with someone. "Compassion is when you feel the pain but don't come up with easy answers. It's what I'd want, someone to feel the pain with me, sit with me and not come up with easy answers."

Commiseration

After she was diagnosed with a rare and supposedly incurable form of cancer, Talia Abramson's closest friend offered her easy answers.

An art curator in New York City who jogged five miles the day she was diagnosed, Talia had come to expect success. But when she learned that a year and a half is considered a long survival time for her disease, she realized she might not see her high school-aged son complete his first year of college. (Note: She did!)

"People think I'll be fine, and they say so," she told me over the phone. "It really upsets me, even when other cancer patients say that. How the hell do you know?"

It upset her even more when one of her best friends tried to reassure her.

"She seems to think part of being a friend is thinking it'll be okay. If she would just commiserate, it would help. Don't fix or deny my pain. Just let me feel it," Talia said.

Allowing a loved one to feel their pain, and feeling their pain with them, can be very frightening. But as physician, cancer support group leader, and author Jeff Kane emphasizes, you don't have to let someone else's pain damage you. You can experience it and then "exhale it out," meaning, just let it go.

But some caregivers and friends cannot release the pain they have taken in because they want to *control* it. They want to make their friend's pain go away. Though no one can make someone else's pain disappear, you can make it more bearable by simply opening yourself to the others' feelings.

We could be in the same boat

Lana was diagnosed with breast cancer after recently moving to the West Coast from the East Coast. Most of her friends were still back East; one, whom Lana described as an Ivy Leaguer, told her via telephone and email what she should do to fight the disease. But Lana is a nurse, and her friend is an attorney.

"Why do you think you have advice to give me?" Lana asked me, as if I were the friend. "I can't really figure this out, but she's four years older than me, and I think she feels a little out of balance in her life right now. And this is her way to try and regain it, to get it under control. But I find it extremely irritating. So I simply don't respond to her messages."

Part of compassion is realizing that you could be going through the same thing—if not the same disease, then the same feeling of imminent disaster, pain, or even death. Compassion is not judgment or condescension.

Merriam-Webster's defines condescension as "voluntary descent from one's rank or dignity in relations with an inferior." But I heard another definition that makes more sense to me: "Condescension is when someone is better off than you, and they know it."

Nancy, a friend of mine who offered us her country home when I was recovering from cancer, shared a story she heard from her boss about the sister of a friend who was dying from breast cancer at age thirty-four.

"A clueless visitor to the house looked over at the girl in bed and said, 'Thank goodness I always ate a healthy diet and got plenty of exercise. This could never happen to me.'"

Nancy continued, "I don't think there's always a reason why bad things happen. 'Why me?' might as well be 'Why not?'"

Fact is, we are all in the same boat. "Life is getting on a boat going out to sea that is going to sink," wrote Pema Chödrön. There are people who smoke three packs a day their whole life and then die at ninety-five after slipping on an icy sidewalk. And there are young women who never smoke nor ever live with a smoker who die at thirty-two of lung cancer. There will be vegetarians who die of colon cancer; meat eaters whose hearts tick until they're a century old; and heavy drinkers whose livers will remain, as long as they live, deep red and fully functioning.

But no one (as far as we know) will live forever. And no one will leave without experiencing some pain. Most of us don't know when or how it will afflict us or whether we will survive it.

Only when we can face and accept these givens—truly accept them—can we feel compassion.

Again, that golden rule

In Buddhism, the first noble truth is "Life is suffering." M. Scott Peck begins his classic, *The Road Less Traveled,* with "Life is difficult." And as the Golden Rule states, "Do unto others as you would have them do unto you." In other words, put yourself in their shoes. Connect with their thoughts and feelings. Realize that it really could be you mourning the loss of your breast, the loss of your illusion of immortality or the possibility of enjoying your own retirement party.

Compassion can be remarkably healing. When you walk even a short distance in a cancer patient's shoes, you often realize how much better your own shoes fit, even if they seemed uncomfortable before. It feels so good when you take the patient's shoes off and slip back into to your old comfortable shoes, which fit you and only you, molding to each of your toes, arches, heels.

I remember comforting my friend Missy when she was fighting colon cancer. No one could have had more to live for: her seven-year-old daughter, Emily, her nine-year-old son, Chris, and her husband, Den, who loved and respected her as much as life itself. She did everything she possibly could do to survive: took a panoply of supplements and tried numerous alternative therapies after chemotherapy failed; prayed and went to church with love, hope, fervor and deep faith; and exercised as best she could. The one thing she could not do was practice visualization.

She had heard again and again that she would enhance her immune system's ability to battle the cancer cells if she could close her eyes and imagine the killer white cells as the little blue monsters in Pac-Man, chasing after the yellow-dot cancer cells and destroying them.

But she just could not do it. She tried visualizing armies; she conjured cells within her body. She read books and tried all the suggested ways to practice therapeutic visualization. But she was not a visual learner. She had a quick mind, a keen sense of humor and compassion, and an immense intellectual and emotional intelligence. But she was opposed to violence, and in spite of having great powers of concentration, she could not picture her cells battling the monsters.

"It was such a scary period of my life. I sometimes felt like I had to be strong and keep up a good face because I didn't want people to feel sorry for me. At times, I wish I could've let others know how bad I really felt."

—D.N., endometrial cancer survivor

"Why can't I do this?" she would ask me.

"Don't sweat it," I'd reply. "Different techniques work for different people. You're doing all sorts of other things that are keeping you strong and healthy. You're doing a superb job." (Now I would say something different, like, "I am so sorry about how you're feeling. It must be scary to think there's more you could be doing to help yourself. I think you are doing a terrific job. I am here for you all the way. Would you like me to do more research into visualization or alternatives for you?")

I watched Missy despair for so long, and I shared her anguish because I had never been able to meditate, in spite of trying at least a half dozen times. If only I had persisted. I wished I had been able to help her by teaching her how to meditate.

I wish I had read *Fighting Cancer from Within* when Missy was sick. The author, Martin Rossman, MD, known internationally as a pioneer in the field of guided imagery, emphasizes not only healing patients, but helping them learn how to help themselves. As he said at the 2004 Cancer as a Turning Point conference in Seattle, "[Visualization] doesn't have to be about fighting. There are many ways to imagine healing. It doesn't have to be about gobbling cancer cells during radiation or having chemotherapy poison them. People can also visualize a healing light or a healing love or a healing of the whole person."

I had so much compassion for Missy when I was diagnosed with cancer myself and felt the pressure upon my own psyche and soul to meditate, to take care of myself in that way. Fortunately, I heeded Dr. Rossman's advice, and I was able to come up with a visualization that suited me perfectly: I imagined my pointy-nosed tan-and-white dog, Bean, who loves to lick (as terriers do), happily lapping up any microscopic cancer cells that remained in my lungs and throughout my body.

Advice separates

Any kind of advice, good or bad, can be more hurtful than helpful, especially if you do not know what it feels like to walk in the other person's shoes.

"As a cancer patient, I would never accept any advice from someone who hasn't had cancer," said therapist Halina Irving, who has been running support groups for people with cancer for two decades. "I don't believe in advice whether we're sick or not without first asking permission to give advice. I believe that as important as human connections are, our autonomy—our entitlement to our own thoughts and feelings and judgment—is also crucially important."

Irving said some people want to give advice because they like the superior position of knowing something, which makes the recipient of the advice feel put down. "But some people want to give advice because they really think they have something of value to impart," she added. Even they should first ask before offering. She suggested we say, "I have some thoughts about what you're going through. Would you like to hear them? My feelings will not be hurt if you'd rather not hear it."

Irving said, as a cancer patient, it's easier to accept advice from someone who has had cancer, but when she runs support groups she always emphasizes that the group's goal is not to advise. "This is about sharing our own experiences," she tells participants, "and as you express your own experience, someone else might find something useful in it, something that we haven't thought of."

She also emphasized that just because a person has had cancer doesn't mean that what worked for him or her will work for someone else. Breast Cancer Action Executive Director Barbara Brenner agrees. "The thing I hated the most was people offering me their treatment-based advice based on what they had done. Phenomenally unuseful."

"I don't like it when anyone starts a sentence with 'you have to.' I LOATH people telling me about alternative medicine or giving me any unsolicited medical advice."

—M.L., pituitary tumor survivor

Soon after I was diagnosed, I was offered advice by a lung cancer survivor whose words terrified and haunted me. Although he was trying to be helpful, his advice was based on his own diagnosis, which was different from mine.

"You really should get a brain scan, because lung cancer can spread to the brain," he told me over the telephone. "I got one, and they found a tumor and took it out right away and I'm fine now."

"But my tumor is really small, and my bone scan was clear," I insisted.

After my tumor was removed and doctors found no cancer cells in my lymph nodes, the man continued to call me; he again inquired about a brain scan.

"There's no reason to believe it has spread to my brain," I said, but his words were now tattooed on my thalamus. It was horrible. I had just gotten out of the hospital after a major surgery; I had spent the previous month in clinics and hospitals getting a PET, CT, and bone scan, a colonoscopy, an ultrasound, and innumerable blood and pulmonary tests. Each one terrified me, and I needed a break.

Finally, I emailed this man whom I had never met and told him he was scaring me and not to call anymore. But it took all my strength because I was so vulnerable, so weak and depressed. And still, his words nagged at me.

I decided the only way to exorcise his advice was to take it.

I had to wait several weeks for the MRI, during which time I suffered headaches (likely psychosomatic) and imagined tumors pressing against my memory center (the memory loss probably had more to do with menopause).

I was fine.

12.

"I am more than my cancer; treat me kindly, not differently."

The whole is more than the sum of its parts.

—Aristotle

ALL OF US PLAY NUMEROUS ROLES in life, as parents, partners, children, colleagues, collectors, music lovers, leaders, friends, foes, and fashion fans—sometimes all at the same time. But when you are diagnosed with cancer, those identities vanish behind the one that eclipses them all: cancer patient.

When my doctor told me I had cancer, everything that had been most important to me (except my family) instantly took a backseat. My career seemed trivial, even though just days before I had beamed with pride at a recent success. Now, if my life were going to end, I would need to accomplish much, much more in order to feel like I had paid my rent on the planet.

I could no longer think of myself as a working writer, producer, media consultant, mother, or even wife. I had cancer, and cancer had me.

I mourned the loss of who I had been. I mourned the loss of my innocence, which shattered abruptly when I realized I could no longer pretend I would live forever. It sounds ridiculous, but most of us live in denial of the fact that we will, indeed, die.

"It's the primordial fear of death and annihilation," explained therapist

Halina Irving. "We're born with that fear, and in our infancy and early childhood, by being nurtured and taken care of by our mothers and by caretakers, we develop denial in the positive sense."

Irving said we have a basic trust that we will not be annihilated, that the environment will provide us with what we need for survival. All that denial builds up over the years until life feels safe. "Always, we think death could happen to someone else and not to me," smiled Irving.

But when someone is diagnosed with cancer, all that denial shatters, and he or she experiences that primordial fear of death.

It changed me in a way I find impossible to explain. I could no longer look in the mirror and imagine the woman I had been before. But even though I could neither see nor be the old me, I did not want to be treated differently. I did not want to be "poor Lori." I just wanted to be "Lori who needs to be treated with a little extra kindness because she has been badly scorched and stands exposed and vulnerable."

Even after a cancer patient's emotional skin reforms to once again protect the nerves beneath, he or she wants to be treated like the same old person. I wanted to be "Good old Lori," just as John Taylor wanted to be known as "Pilot John."

> *"Overall, I felt like I developed a new reputation in my small communities of faith and family as 'someone one with breast cancer.' For about a year, pretty much every conversation began (and some STILL DO!) with an earnest inquiry: 'How are you feeling?' I know they meant well. But relying on my partner to convey info about my health was an enormous relief!"*
>
> —S.D., breast cancer survivor

"I want to be at the controls"

Even before John Taylor could read, his two most prized possessions were books: one was about taking a trip on a passenger plane, the other, a children's encyclopedia that included illustrations of a pilot flying an airplane: "Push the wheel, houses get bigger. Pull the wheel, houses get smaller," John remembered hearing his mother read to him. "Those words and seeing the movie *Airport* on TV fueled a vivid fantasy of me being 'The Kid Who Saved That Jetliner by Taking the Controls when the Pilots Ate the Bad Fish.'"

What finally propelled John to learn how to fly was a summer class about airplanes that he took at a local museum when he was twelve. "It concluded with a flight up front in a real airplane, a Beechcraft V35 Bonanza, and I got to try my hand at the controls. Sure enough, I pushed the yoke and the houses got bigger. I pulled the yoke back and the houses got smaller. I was hooked!"

Never one to shy away from a challenge, John learned to pilot a plane at a tiny two-thousand-foot strip with trees in the approach path; though he was working full-time, he always made time to fly.

Getting his Private Pilot Certificate took seventy-two hours over nine months, flying once or twice a week, and about five thousand dollars. He will never forget the day of his first solo (a banner day for every pilot).

He fell deeply in love with flying and the freedom it afforded. I understood, because I had become a pilot in my twenties, and it had both lifted my confidence and given me the freedom to come back down to earth after a wild ride of indecision about my career.

John loved the mental as well as the physical freedom. "Being able to move around in all three dimensions, unobstructed, and above a carpet of beautiful scenery is always liberating. Liberating mentally, too. Because flying safely takes 100 percent of your concentration and attention, all your outside worries disappear."

But while his spirits had been soaring, his body had been secretly spiraling downwards. His lymph nodes had slowly swelled until they had reached the size of peach pits. John went to the doctor, and less than a month after getting his pilot license, he learned he had Hodgkin's lymphoma.

"Okay, now the real adventure begins," he remembered thinking. He had every possible medical test to determine the stage of his illness, which would determine his treatment. But finally he had to have the enlarged lymph node in his neck removed. He was awake during the procedure because his insurance would not pay for general anesthesia.

"Some people refused to talk to me when I got sick. They looked at my mother, my sister, or my doctor but rarely, if ever, made eye contact with me."

—D.S., neuroblastoma survivor

What jarred him most during the operation was hearing the doctors' surprise as they removed the largest node. "They dropped it into the cocktail cup and said, 'You just won the Olympics of lymph nodes.' I said, 'You mean the O*lymph*ics?'"

John's sense of humor faded as complications from his surgery set in. He had horrible cramping in his abdomen and had to have another operation to cut the membrane that contained his intestines. They cut the nerves of his prostate plexus by mistake, so he could no longer ejaculate. Though he could still enjoy orgasm, he would not be able to have children. He had wanted to teach his own children to fly some day.

"I didn't want to be treated any differently, which is why I decided to wear a wig so no one would know about my ongoing treatment unless I chose to tell them."

—R.L., breast cancer survivor

John continued to pilot an airplane throughout his chemotherapy and radiation.

"During my treatment I used to fly (always with an instructor aboard), and from the minute I took off until a good three hours after I landed, it was the only time I was totally pain free."

The second most-painful part of his cancer experience was the way people behaved around him. Although his boss did not treat him differently and never called attention to his illness, his family did.

"I needed to do certain things for myself. I wanted to cook for myself, and I wanted to play tennis. My dad came to visit and was trying to cook for me and everything. Finally I had to tell him to go home."

Always independent, John said his father's solicitude made him feel like he was different from and "less than" his peers. Once he was free of his father and others who continued to coddle him and treat him like a patient, he was able to feel normal again and resume his old life, which included flying solo.

"Surviving cancer just reinforced the great feelings I already had about flying. I think flying actually changed my feelings about cancer more than vice versa. Learning to fly is an often daunting and discouraging task that requires lots of effort and study and transforming self-doubt into self-confidence. It's all driven by hope, survival instinct, personal drive, encouragement from others, and perseverance toward a goal. When it came to fighting cancer, I'd already been through the drill."

"I am not what I eat"

Talia did everything right when her friend, Monica Schneider, was sick with cancer. "She set up an email list to send out bulletins to let people know what was going on with me so I didn't have to do it," Monica told me over the phone. "She also made a sign for my door when I was going through chemo. My immune system was suppressed, and I had to be protected from certain things. The sign had seventy-two items on it saying 'No cold, no flu, no bronchitis, no elephantiasis . . .' So that was pretty amusing."

Talia did almost everything a great pal is supposed to do, except stay with Monica. The night before I was to interview Monica, Talia died of a heart attack.

I knew Talia had died because I read about it in the newspaper. A high-profile activist in the Bay Area, Talia had created an online newsletter that pricked many a local politician whose activities and ethics she questioned—and who publicly admitted that they would miss her sorely.

I knew Monica was Talia's friend because the article quoted Monica. Immediately, I picked up the phone and left Monica a brief voicemail expressing my sympathy and saying I would call her to reschedule our interview in a couple of weeks.

When the day of the interview arrived a month later, the first subject we discussed was Talia and her sudden death. "She was in the kitchen making a cup of tea and just died. Her heart and lungs just stopped," Monica said. "We knew she might not live to a ripe old age because she had congestive heart disease, but it's still such a shock."

I didn't know what to say, so I tried to practice what cancer survivors had been advising during my research. "I'm so sorry," I said, and let her talk. Soon she turned the subject to her own illness and the subject of this book.

"I went in with a list of weird symptoms," Monica began. "I had night sweats, my ears were stopped up after I gave lectures, and I had a lump on the left side of my rib cage. I told the doctor I was going into menopause."

He irrigated her ears and sent her off for a CT scan and an ultrasound. "I had a sneaking suspicion something was seriously wrong. I had a persistent cough. I just knew on some level, and I actually made peace with the idea that I might have cancer and I might die."

Monica wasn't going to die. She had a highly treatable case of non-Hodgkin's lymphoma. She would, however, need chemotherapy.

Single and fiercely independent, Monica knew what she wanted. She wanted to live, and she wanted to live the way *she* wanted. Although she wanted help with certain chores, she wanted to maintain control as she always had over what she ate and how she lived.

"I'm a picky eater anyway, and my sister and friends would shop for me. I'd make a very specific list—'I want Campbell's Bean with Bacon soup.' They'd either come back with the generic brand or give me flak about my food preferences. 'If I want to eat Hostess Twinkies, well, if it will get me through cancer, I'll eat them!' I would say. I had a friend with cancer who had been avoiding nitrites her whole life, and she said, 'I have cancer now so let's have some bacon!'"

Monica likes it when people show they care, but she prefers that they treat her the way they always have and not handle her with kid gloves. (Some people like to be treated with kid gloves, but if you don them, it is best to wear them invisibly. See chapter 15, "My moods change day to day; please forgive me if I snap at you.")

Then Monica chuckled. "My cousin kept saying 'Eat green, leafy vegetables; get a blender and make smoothies.' And when I wasn't doing that, I was supposed to visualize green, leafy vegetables. 'Want me to bring you a chard milkshake?' she asked me."

People gave Monica books and printouts about various risk factors and even her five-year survival rate. She threw it all in the recycling bin. "I didn't want that information. And people gave me tapes—meditation tapes. I never did any of that shit. I wrote a book instead. I wrote *This Is What I Did on My Cancer Vacation*."

One thing Monica really wanted to do during her "cancer vacation" was attend a professional conference she had been looking forward to for months. It was to be held shortly after she had completed chemotherapy. Some of her friends urged her not to go because she would have to fly on an airplane and expose herself to germs.

"Treat us like we are still normal. We may be sick, or we may have been ill, but we are still the same people we were before cancer. Don't look at us with pity in your eyes or voice. Don't be patronizing."

—D.F., prostate cancer survivor

"Sometimes you just want to forget and not be the patient," she said, suddenly serious. "One of the reasons I wanted to go to the conference was so I could just be a person. I went there and no one said, 'It's 1 A.M., shouldn't you be going to bed now?' I got to be a regular person."

It's been three years since Monica's diagnosis. "When I get to five years, I'll be considered 'cured.' So I'm going to have a party and serve only cured foods—olives and ham and the like!"

Even if you are "cured," many people still think of you as a cancer survivor.

When my cousin Barbara reached her five-year mark, she no longer chose to call herself a cancer survivor. "I've had many things happen in my past that I don't identify myself in terms of because they're no longer part of me," she wrote, "and cancer is one such thing. For example, I'm divorced, but I don't consider myself a divorcée. I had measles, but I don't consider myself a measles survivor. I used to be a waitress, but I don't consider myself an ex-waitress."

"It was important to me that people realize that I had a small cancerous tumor in one breast, that was all. I regret that we become defined by that one element. The rest of me was damn healthy! In fact, I told the surgeon that he must have made a mistake."

—N.E., breast cancer survivor

But shaking the label of waitress or divorcée is easier than changing your reputation as a cancer survivor. A stigma often persists, making the disease more powerful than it should be, especially when someone is still fighting it.

"They have a disease, but they're still the same person, and to change the way you react to that person makes the disease more important than what attracted you to that person in the first place," observed Bay Area Tumor Institute Executive Director Barry Siegel.

Physician-turned-support-group leader Jeff Kane urges caregivers to see the whole person, not just his or her illness. In *How to Heal: A Guide for Caregivers,* he wrote: "We need to accept the sick person without applying judgments about his physical condition, his prognosis, our contact with him, or its outcome.

"To the extent we see the sick person as a 'patient,' we'll relate to his patienthood instead of his wider identity," continued Kane. "In particular, we'll undervalue his strengths. While he's sick, remember, he's unusually vulnerable to the opinions of others, so if we see him as a helpless victim, he's likely to see himself that way, too."

Judy Larsen not only felt like a victim, she wondered whether she had given herself cancer. Uterine cancer is hormone-induced, and she had taken hormones. She, like many cancer patients, took responsibility for something that is an act of science or nature, not of self or God.

Six days after surgery, she had enough energy to go out for a couple of hours, so she asked a friend to take her to a yarn store. "I wanted to knit something for each member of my family before I died," she wrote. (This was eleven years ago!)

Her friend knew it was a bit too soon for an outing, but took her anyway.

"There were no negative comments about feelings. She said, 'Okay, when do you want to go?' She helped me look for yarn and choose it and acted as if we were having fun. I really couldn't decide on much and got very tired. After a bit, she helped me get back to the car. She never told me I should not be out or up or that I wasn't going to die."

Judy's friend saw and accepted Judy as herself, as the friend she knew and enjoyed. She allowed Judy the freedom to see herself as a cancer victim, but also to reach beyond that. By showing such love, Judy's friend helped her live.

13.

"I want you to help without my asking you to."

Say yes when nobody asked.

—Lao proverb

I HAD JUST BEEN DIAGNOSED with lung cancer. Although I gave up my writing and consulting work, I became busier than ever. My time was no longer filled by the luxuries and exigencies of work, grocery shopping, haircuts, meal preparation, or making love. Welcome to Cancerland, where research, conversation, doctors' appointments, and medical tests fill most every moment.

I had just had a PET, or positron emission tomography, scan to see whether there were signs of cancer outside my lungs. PET scans show sugars metabolized in the body. Since cancer causes a higher rate of caloric burning (hence the weight loss associated with the disease), affected areas show up on the colorful scanned images.

The day after the PET scan, I decided to take a break to have my bangs trimmed. I sat in a brown vinyl swivel chair, watching protectively as a stylist ran her special thinning scissors through my hair. I was afraid she would cut my bangs short, making my face looking like a pixie's. Of course my fear was magnified, as I was awaiting test results and was extremely anxious and vulnerable.

I had told the stylist that I had cancer and was soon going in for major surgery. She had shaken her head with a "tsk-tsk."

When my cell phone rang, my hand bolted to the counter two feet in front of me and pushed the call button before the phone could ring a second time. What I heard turned my face white; it was fight or flight time. "Baboom! Baboom! Baboom!" cried my heart.

> *"My friend said, 'If you need anything—someone to clean toilets or to punch around to blow off stress—I'm available from 9 to 9:15 this Tuesday.' It made me feel like laughing, because it was an offer, but I didn't have to make a real commitment. She was there if I needed her, but she wouldn't be hurt if I didn't."*
>
> —S.M., uterine cancer survivor

"Lori, there are several areas of your PET scan that show increased metabolic activity," my surgeon said.

"Where?" I demanded.

"In your abdominal area."

I felt the heat of tears in my eyes. "What does that mean? Has the cancer spread?"

"Not necessarily. You need to come in, and we need to talk about this," he replied calmly.

"But I need to know!"

"This is not something we should talk about over the phone," he insisted.

"But . . . but . . ." Heavy breathing. *Deep breaths, Lori,* I told myself. "Okay," I surrendered, too weak to challenge the man who was hopefully going to help save my life.

"Can you come in tomorrow morning at ten?" he asked.

I hung up the phone and wanted to scream. Instead, I asked what I owed the stylist for the three-minute thinning she had yet to finish.

"Five dollars," she replied.

I rummaged through my purse for my wallet, but I was shaking so much I kept losing my grip. The stylist waited silently. I finally grabbed the billfold and pulled out a crisp five.

Walking home from my appointment, my mind was a washing machine spinning through cycles of worry, dread, and anger. If the stylist had said, "Don't worry about paying, it's okay . . ." or, "I'm so sorry; it sounds like you got some bad news," I would have felt less polluted, less marked with a giant "C."

I was vulnerable, desperately in need of nurturing, kindness, and comfort. "May I give you a hug?" would have meant the world to me. Instead I heard, "Five dollars."

She meant no harm, I know that. She had absolutely no idea how I was feeling or what I needed. She was shocked and scared herself, I'm sure. But, still, she blew it. She blew an opportunity to make a difference.

I would not have asked her to waive her fee, but if she had thought to offer that, it would have made an impression I could take to my grave (some distant day).

If she had treated me with kid gloves—without letting me know it, that is—I would have repaid her with lifelong love, respect, and admiration.

The gift of work

I heard about a form of aid that touched me deeply. It was a gift of dignity and identity, a gift that not only helped a woman in the short-term but helped give her a long life, enabling her to see grandchildren she never expected she would live to love.

Virginia Mei reached halfway across the world, sifting through more than a half century of memories, to recall the day in her homeland of China that the Red Guard came to her door and demanded her bible. She was barely eighteen.

"I was frightened. Had to let them in, give our bible." She had stepped aside to let three young men climb the narrow stairway to her family's second-floor apartment.

"The word of Mao was the word of God," she recalled, her mind in China but her body in San Francisco, weaving effortlessly through the tourists and Asian Americans moving along the Chinatown sidewalk.

Though she was shorter than I, I had to hasten my pace to keep up with the sixty-eight-year-old. Brocaded silk robes of bright purple, azure, green, scarlet, and red hung from metal dress racks and shined in the midafternoon spotlight of early winter. The

"A friend's teen-aged daughters planted flowers in my garden without my asking. They were beautiful!"

—A.T., ovarian cancer survivor

sun's heat released the fragrance of bananas and persimmons stacked high on produce stands. But my senses were drawn to Virginia, as her memories came to life in my mind. I imagined her standing in her doorway in 1953, the year of my birth, watching lean uniformed young men climb her stairs in an attempt to rob her of her unflappable faith in God.

"I was a medical doctor in China," she continued, as we sat across from one another in her small rectangular office with a window looking out on the steel blue bay. Though she had been trained in one of the world's most prestigious professions, she displayed great humility and warmth.

> *"I loved it when friends would call each other about what I needed instead of me having to make the phone call when I felt so terrible. Wow, I had incredible friends!"*
>
> —S.R., skin cancer survivor

"Oh, I'm so proud to have you interview me, a medical journalist! And you are a cancer survivor, you got lung cancer, two years ago?" she probed gently. A caregiver by nature, it was difficult for her to turn her attention back to herself.

"I have my college education in the 1950s and '60s in Mainland China," she explained. "Students took only one class in school, learning Mao's theories and ideas. If you had any problems or difficulties, you were expected to consult a party member. What Chairman Mao would do, you follow. It was very ridiculous in several respects."

Virginia left the party and China after practicing medicine there for fifteen years. She traveled to the United States to help support her son and to pursue a life where she was free to worship the God she still loved. Her husband would follow as soon as he could get a visa, but for the time, she was on her own.

Virginia's cousin, a publisher of a local bilingual Chinese American newspaper, hired her as an editor. Although her English was very limited, she had a brilliant command of the Chinese language, and though she missed the healing profession, she loved being so closely linked to her community.

She became comfortable in her new home, living with her son and earning money to help with his college tuition at UC Berkeley. She worked many hours.

"I'm so busy that I don't feel that I'm sick. But in my bowels, there was a little bit of fresh blood." She thought it might be hemorrhoids. "But deep down in my heart, because I am a medical doctor," she admitted, "I have this alert that maybe it is or maybe not hemorrhoid, but in my heart I am struggling."

Virginia lived with that struggle for too long, she said. By the time she sought medical attention, the tumor had grown to 4½ centimeters.

"I have to blame myself because I did not go to the doctor," she said angrily. Heaped on top of her self-blame was terrible fear and loneliness.

"It was all kept inside. Because I was living with my son. He was so busy studying, so I don't want to bother him. I don't want to upset my son and my good friends."

Although Virginia did tell her husband, he was still in China and was unable to enter the United States because he couldn't get a visa. The only others she told were her pastor and his wife.

"I don't want to make it spread out, because I myself am suffering. I have to—how you say—adjust myself and I had to think correctly. Too many things."

The stigma of cancer, pervasive in her community, oppressed her, too. It was like living under Communist rule. "Especially in Chinatown, there are some people, they're not well-educated, so they don't understand about cancer. They only know this is a very serious disease.

"Some people think that it is bad luck, it is contagious. So people just keep the distance. And also, some people just feel that, 'Oh, maybe you've done something very bad and then you got punished.' This was twenty years ago. It was so bad."

As an educated woman and a medical professional, Virginia did not blame herself for getting cancer and, of course, knew she wasn't contagious. But the knowledge she had, as a doctor, made her fear other things. She finally told her son about her disease.

"My life expectancy was very low. I wondered, how long can I live?"

Doctors operated on Virginia for eight and a half hours, removing her colon and performing a colostomy, an operation that creates an artificial anus through an opening made in the abdomen. It was difficult adjusting to the pouch she carries with her always.

"At the very beginning you don't get used to it, and you're scared to go into public. Sometimes you'd get a leak, so there is that smell. And that makes you very, very nervous. I don't want to bother people. But things have improved and improved. And I have adjusted."

Another adjustment would be just as difficult. At forty-eight, she had worked for almost three decades as a physician and later an editor, and she was accustomed to feeling useful and of value. Without a job to give her a sense of purpose and keep her occupied, she fell into a depression. Luckily, there was someone there to offer her something that gave her one more reason to live. It was her pastor, Ernest Woo, one of the three people she had told of her cancer.

Woo called and said he wanted to see Virginia. She thought he wanted to visit, that the call was a courtesy call. "But he comes to me and says, 'I have a job for you, and I hope you can come and help.' I never looked for this job. I never looked for it," she smiled, shaking her soft gray hair and wiping tears from her eyes.

"I needed to hear my friends say, 'I'm bringing over dinner,' without asking me if I wanted them to make dinner or what I wanted to eat. Hell, I didn't know what I wanted to eat. I had bigger problems than food!"

—S.N., lung cancer survivor

Woo was not only a pastor, but a family and marriage counselor, and he was working at a neighborhood clinic in Chinatown.

Virginia giggled with glee. "He said, 'Look, come and help me.' I felt very grateful! It was a compliment!" Though she did not have a degree in counseling, she had received some training in mental health because she was an MD in China. Even so, she told Woo that she worried she might not live long.

That did not faze him. He told her to think about it, and he'd come back to see her in a week.

"I just put it in my prayers," she smiled. "And I talk to my son, and he said, 'Look, Mom, this is part-time.' He knows that inside my mind is not so—how do you say—balanced or peaceful. He feels that. And then he says, 'You need to go out and have some work and see people every day; it's good for you!'"

Slowly, because she was still recovering from surgery, Virginia trained with her new mentor. Though she knew little about counseling, she understood suffering, and she quickly learned how to assuage it. Speaking three different dialects of Chinese—Cantonese, Mandarin, and Shanghai—she has enlarged her client base, counseling men, women, and youth from her homeland who need help coping with family or marriage problems.

A few years ago, Virginia read a column in a Chinese newspaper written by a woman who got breast cancer and underwent surgery, radiation, and chemotherapy alone. After Virginia got well, she wondered, *How come we Chinese people don't help each other?*

That inspired her to start an ongoing cancer support group for Chinese American women. Though short-term groups existed to help them through their crises, there was nothing ongoing to help reduce the stigma of cancer and increase the sense of community so vital to good mental health.

"We want to educate our people that this is just like high blood pressure or diabetes. Everyone has a chance to survive. This is no punishment. We like to have people walking with us through this difficulty. Come walk beside me!"

It is hard to imagine anyone who feels healthier than Dr. Mei, and I can't help but believe a huge part of the credit belongs to Woo. The help he gave her, without her having to ask—the gift he knew she needed by listening to her and understanding her history and her hopes—has spread to the hundreds she has counseled during the last eighteen years.

"How can I help?"

Although most people appreciate being helped without having to ask, there are times when doing so can backfire. A neighbor emailed me an example as unusual as it is puzzling and disturbing.

"Here's the story of my blunder," she began.

"My colleague, a former reporter named Mary, was writing speeches when she was diagnosed with stage 3 breast cancer at age forty-four. She and her husband had gone to Peru four years earlier to adopt a Peruvian infant when he was just a few weeks old." The baby fulfilled the couple's longtime dream.

When Mary learned she had cancer, she thought she had been sentenced to death. "And so there she was; with eleven lymph nodes involved, she was a candidate for a bone marrow transplant," the neighbor wrote. The transplant extended Mary's life by a few months, during which time she came into the office to work as often as she could.

When Mary's cancer reappeared in her

"Someone with cancer is too overwhelmed, tired, or sick to reach out and call people to ask for help. Friends should call the patient, and ask when the next doctor's appointment is, and offer to drive the patient or sit with them during chemo."

—J.D., breast cancer survivor

bones, my neighbor and her colleagues wanted to help by organizing shifts of people to clean her house, help with child care, shop, and cook.

My neighbor was designated the one to offer their services. She was completely unprepared for Mary's response. "She wanted nothing from us; she was insulted and furious. 'I can pay someone to clean my house,' she said. 'I know you want to help, but I can't take care of your needs. I'm looking at the last year of my life, and I'm leaving a five-year-old.'"

My neighbor felt horrible. "To have approached Mary full of love and to have made her feel worse was devastating. Over time I have come to understand her response, I think; perhaps when people are dying, one of the things they must cope with is being totally out of control. . . . Rejecting our offer and arranging for her own help might have given her back some control and dignity.

"I think she was so angry at dying, so grief stricken at leaving her son, that there was nothing we could do for her. Maybe sometimes there is no comfort that can come from the outside," my neighbor concluded.

Although that may seem true at times, there is one thing that almost always brings comfort, and you needn't ask permission to give it: Silently sending love, or praying, has never been shown to cause harm and has actually been shown to improve health.

14.

"I like to be held in your thoughts or prayers."

Prayer doesn't change things; it changes people, and they change things.

—Anonymous

ARTIE GOLDEN SUSPECTED A bladder infection when he found himself both needing to urinate frequently (not uncommon for a man of sixty-three) and experiencing a burning sensation while doing so. His doctor put him on antibiotics, but when the second regimen failed, he consulted a urologist.

After a battery of tests, Artie was diagnosed with bladder cancer. He had no tumors and therefore didn't warrant surgery. Instead, he underwent an unusual treatment. Although it was more than six years ago, Artie can recount almost every detail.

"I got this live tuberculin bacillus injected into my bladder each week," he began, as if telling a mystery story. "The bladder detects a substance and tries to slough off cells. They put 50 ccs into the bladder, and then have you lay on your left side fifteen minutes, then your right side, then your back and front, swishing it around."

I pictured mouthwash, then a Pepto Bismol commercial; then I saw myself pouring oil into a baking dish, tilting it back and forth to prep it for oven-roasted vegetables. I was fascinated that such a high-tech treatment relies on something as basic as gravity.

Artie continued, "You go home and hold it for one hour, and then urinate." I flashed back to getting a pelvic ultrasound exam after my positive PET scan and having to endure a full bladder while the tech probed me to find another tumor—possibly multiple ones.

"Then you treat the toilet with Clorox. There's a cure rate of 80 percent . . . and I had great results," he sighed, "except in one spot."

He needed an eight-and-a-half hour operation to remove the remaining cancer. "They took out my bladder and prostate and transected my urethra—and for fun they took out the appendix," he laughed.

"It was 100 percent successful. They make a bladder out of your bowel, take it out, and filet it so they can reconnect it. But my surgeon couldn't reconnect it, so I have to use a catheter every four to six hours to urinate.

"You lose your sexual function," he said matter-of-factly. "You have to live with that. Attitude is a big part of it. If you have a positive attitude, that's as good as any medicine they can give you. Let's go forward with life."

One thing that helped him move forward was the tremendous outpouring of love and support he received from his family and his religious congregation. Though not "overly religious," he believes prayer helped him heal.

"There must be some power greater than what I can discern. I went to a Bar Mitzvah a few months ago, and I ran into a casual friend who's also a cancer survivor. He said to me, 'I come to the temple every morning and I pray for you every day.'" Artie paused. "Even now—still—six years later, he's praying for me every day! It makes you feel so great. And I really believe that has helped me survive."

The power of believing in someone

Belief is crucial; soon after Carol's diagnosis, belief was almost everything. She emailed practically everyone on her address list, requesting they send good thoughts or prayers her way. She knew she needed all the support she could get, and she felt no shame in asking for it.

She received hundreds of emails, phone calls, and greeting cards from friends, acquaintances, colleagues, and even friends of friends. All assured and buoyed her spirits and hopes, except for one person.

"An old friend from grade school, Brandon, emailed me and said he wasn't going to pray for me because he didn't believe prayer was effective. He was a microbiologist," Carol added, "and he did say he would send all love my way."

He also sent a fabulous bouquet of two dozen white lilies with bright orange stamens. "Their sweet and very strong fragrance stuck in my nasal hairs—just like his refusal to pray for me stuck in my heart," Carol recalled.

"As much as I appreciated his love and respected his right to his opinion, Brandon's comment pierced me." Like a hypodermic, it spread a dye of doubt. She wanted to believe that all the prayers would make a difference, and even though she believed thought, love, and prayer to be similar in purpose, she also believed there was something more cosmic or real about prayer. She had volunteered at a hospice and had once attended Harvard University School of Continuing Education's "Spirituality and Healing in Medicine" conference with Dr. Herbert Benson. Over the years, she had kept up with the latest on healing. A recent study had shown that patients in a coronary care unit who were prayed for had significantly fewer complications. But another study—the one Carol's grammar school friend cited—had shown prayer had no influence.

"I understood that. With his background, of course Brandon would say that. But that's not what I needed to hear. At that point, I needed all the ammunition I could gather, every force I could bring to bear, not just to fight my cancer but to keep my head and heart above water. I felt like I was sinking."

Like many people who feel particularly vulnerable, Carol also fell victim to superstition. Gandhi said, "Prayers are no superstitions; they are more real than the acts of eating, drinking, sitting, or walking." But to Carol, superstition and prayer went hand in hand. "Even though I don't believe in a thumbs up/thumbs down God with a gray beard who

"I also wanted people to pray for me—I asked EVERYONE to keep me in their prayers, and I feel like it made a huge difference in my outcome!"

—J.M., soft tissue sarcoma survivor

makes decisions on a case-by-case basis, I may have thought of my cancer as an election of sorts. The more votes—meaning the more prayers—the better."

Carol called Brandon to thank him for the beautiful flowers and love he had sent, and then she brought up the subject of prayer. "I thought I was just curious; I respected his opinion, and we had always had interesting conversations about controversial issues. He was one of the brightest, most loving and thoughtful men I'd ever met.

"But," she continued, "I suspect I may have just wanted to be right. I wanted Brandon to agree with me. But he dug in his heels. 'I'm sorry. I just don't believe that prayer can heal people,' he insisted. 'I've read the studies, and they're just not conclusive.'

"What I realized after our conversation was that I not only wanted to believe that prayer works but I wanted him to care enough about me to stretch a little . . . to reach out . . . maybe even to misrepresent his beliefs to me, without lying." She wanted him to treat her with invisible kid gloves.

Perhaps Brandon could have said, "A lot of studies do support that notion."

"Would it have been so hard for him to say that?" Carol asked. "Part of me still feels angry. But the other part knows he loves me. He not only said so, he showed it, over and over, with flowers, greeting cards, and other symbols."

Fact is, when you feel that weak and vulnerable, you do not want conflict. Although Carol did invite it, she wanted Brandon's support. "He undermined my faith, and although I know that was not at all his intention, that was the effect."

Organized prayer

When I had cancer, my cousin Barbara contacted a group of religious women at a convent who agreed to pray for me night and day. My congregation at Alameda's Temple Israel said a *Mi Sheberach* (a traditional healing prayer) every week for me at Friday night services, while my Christian friends offered their own prayers. My nonreligious friends and my medical doctor, a Buddhist, meditated on my healing. My friend Nasús came over and performed a Native American sage smudge on my home to purify it and promote healing. Although I did not know a sage smudge from sandal-wood incense, I could feel the love as surely as I could smell the sweet musky smoke permeating the furniture and walls of my home. The love was visible, and it brought forth tears.

"I don't think it's possible to overrate sick people's need for attention," wrote physician Jeff Kane in *How to Heal: A Guide for Caregivers*. He said people in his cancer support group have been telling him that for years. "When we feel recognized, witnessed, understood, we shine. We feel tangibly better: Recognition is a major healing stimulant, on a par, I'd say, with adequate sleep.

"If closeness promotes healing," he continued, "then we're asking for trouble when we increase distance. As much as sick people love being heard, they get angry when they're not heard."

I told my surgeon that I believe in the power of prayer, and told her I was praying for her and her team and I wanted her to pray, too, if she was comfortable doing so. She said, 'I believe in the power of prayer,' and squeezed my hand. I went into surgery calmly and optimistically."

—M.E., colon cancer survivor

When Brandon argued with Carol, she felt he was putting distance between them. "I needed him to stay close, even though he was thousands of miles away."

But what would have made Carol feel close to Brandon made Peter Dawson feel distant and almost desperate. His mother, Mary, explained. "My daughter-in-law is dying of cancer," she said, pain quieting her voice almost to a whisper. "What she and my son have been going through is so hard. People will look at them and say, 'Well, I'm praying for you.' There's a kind of sense that you're already dead. You don't say to someone who's had a heart attack, 'I'm praying for you.'

"There's an implication here that's very hard to tolerate," Mary continued. "My son told me, 'I thank people, I appreciate their prayers, but I'd probably just rather people say, 'I'm hanging in there for you,' or, 'I'm thinking about you.'"

Mary concluded, almost bitterly, "The prayer thing really smacks of 'You ain't gonna live long.'"

To Mary and her son, it may smack of death because the woman they love is dying of lung cancer and, at this point, there is no hope for a cure.

Even though they may accept that reality, they do not want other people rubbing their face in it.

"I'm praying for you" might mean something altogether different to Mary and Peter once their beloved has died. "And that's one of the problems," said Brother Daniel of the New Camaldoli silent monastery and retreat center. "For people who don't pray much, it can be frightening when they hear that other people are praying for them. Some people associate praying only with funerals. And that's why it scares them."

The monks at New Camaldoli, a haven high on a hill above Central California's rugged coast, pray daily. An integral part of their lives, prayer is, to them, as nourishing as love.

> *"I have a tremendous faith in God, and I really had to keep reminding myself to give it up to the higher power. My friends and family know this and helped me to stay connected to my beliefs."*
>
> —R.Y., kidney cancer survivor

Whether being prayed for improves health or not, virtually everyone appreciates being cared for, thought of, and loved. It may be best to ask permission—"May I pray for you? Would you like that?"—before telling someone you are sending mental telegrams to the Great Upstairs. But if you have love to send, do so. Perhaps it will come back to you someday and help *you* live.

15.
"My moods change day to day; please forgive me if I snap at you."

Some situations are so bad that to remain sane is insane.

—Frederich Nietzsche

EVERYONE HAS MOOD SWINGS, but many of us who have had cancer experience them more frequently and severely. Though we may react one way one day, we might react quite differently to the same words or actions the next day, week, or month.

As oncology social worker Sandy Bezet, who recently had breast cancer herself, told me, "Just because I don't feel like talking today doesn't mean I won't feel like talking tomorrow." She believes friends should check in regularly, but she fears some friends use a no today as an excuse to stay away indefinitely.

"It's an easy out for those of us uncomfortable with emotional feelings. If you say, 'I don't want to talk,' that kind of person will say, 'Well, she said three weeks ago she didn't want to talk, so I'm not going to ask her anymore.'"

Jill Jordan, who was diagnosed with late-stage lung cancer three years ago, said it didn't bother her, during chemotherapy, if someone asked about her plans for the next year. But during other times, it would scare her to think twelve months ahead because she didn't know if she would be alive then.

Personalities can go from Jekyll to Hyde in a matter of seconds. Mine did, especially between my diagnosis and my surgery. When my dad and my stepmom, Judy, came to visit, I felt so shaky, so unnerved, so off the charts, that I knew I had to warn them.

They had just arrived for a three-and-a-half week stay. After only a few minutes of catching up in the kitchen, I told them there was something I wanted to talk to them about. In retrospect, that must have terrified them. But it wasn't them I was thinking about.

"Let's go into the living room," I suggested, and took several deep breaths.

My thoughts and feelings muddled together like colored paints blending to form a dirty brown. I was frightened at what I was about to say; frightened at the depth of my fear. I was frightened that what I was about to say would make my parents stand up and leave the room, leave the state of California, leave me forever.

> "I loved it when my friends and family tolerated my occasional unexpected sarcasm. It wasn't like me to be that way at all, but I wasn't always myself."
>
> —R.R., melanoma survivor

"I am more terrified than I have ever been in my life," I finally revealed. "I don't expect you to understand, because I don't think you really can unless you've been through this. But I am so afraid, I can't even describe it.

"So I want to warn you," I continued, terrified that they would not understand. "I know you might think I'm overly sensitive sometimes, but I'm even more sensitive than ever right now. I may be unpredictable. I may snap at you. I may say things I don't mean. And I just want to tell you that and ask you in advance to forgive me and to step lightly."

The fear on their faces relaxed into relief as they realized I was not going to tell them I had six months to live. My stepmom, Judy, a kind and deeply compassionate individual, said, "Of course," and stood up to give me a hug. Dad did, too, and the three of us shared a moment of love during which I may have forgotten (for about five nanoseconds) that I had cancer.

I don't know how I was able to sit down and speak with Dad and Judy that afternoon. Where did I get the courage? Perhaps it was instinctual—about surviving. Maybe it came from trusting them so much. Whatever inspired me, others may not have the time, opportunity, or inclination to have such conversations with their loved ones. Often people with cancer snap or even blow up without knowing why or before they have a chance to consider that they might transfer their feelings of anger about cancer to whomever or whatever happens to be close by at the time.

Don't give up on us

When Diana Delaney and her fiancé, Baruch, were struggling with the demands and dangers of his numerous surgeries and his rapidly changing state of health, their moods changed rapidly, as well. They had many supporting, loving friends, but how they wanted to interact with them changed frequently.

"Sometimes you want them to call two or three times and check in; sometimes you want them not to call back. I'm thinking of my two best friends," Diana recalled.

"I hope I can come up with as much love as they did if they ever need me in that way. When I was mean, they showed up again the next day. When I was needy and weepy, they were there."

Being there, showing up, means trying again and again when loved ones shut you out.

"You know how some people ask you, 'Do you need so-and-so?'" asked Melissa King, who had been treated for both breast cancer and melanoma. "And so you say, 'I'm taken care of that way, and then they stop asking after that one time? But I had another friend that I'd say no to and she'd still offer because she knew there would come a time when I would accept it.

"She would ask each and every day, 'Do you have someone to take you? Are you eating dinner tonight? Are you taken care of this week?' and I really liked that."

Melissa added that that particular friend had survived cancer herself. Not surprising. People whose loved ones have helped them live know what it takes to help others along the same path of healing.

Psychologist Paul Ekman, whose seminal research on facial expressions and the hundreds of muscles that belie our feelings, said it's important to know who you are dealing with when deciding how assertive to be with a friend.

> *"I just needed them to understand that I was not at my best mentally and emotionally and to be patient with me."*
>
> —T.U., prostate cancer survivor

"I have one friend who is quite a close friend, but he's such a reserved person that I can never expect him to call me when he's ill, even though he's not married and he has no children," Ekman said. "I'm one of the few people, when he gets a treatment and someone has to take him home, that he can ask. There aren't many people like that, but I have to tell him again and again, 'I want to!' because he won't take more initiative."

Taking initiative applies not only to helping the person you care for who has cancer but helping yourself. It is another way to help your loved one live.

Posttreatment depression and anger

A year and a half ago, if you had asked me if I was in remission, I might have started crying. If you had asked to bring a hot meal over, I might also have wept, for an entirely different reason.

Still raw from my diagnosis and surgery, still worried about whether and how I could possibly integrate the experience into my life and "move on," I felt like I had suffered from the worst possible case of premenstrual syndrome. One day I would awaken and shed a few tears of joy and gratitude because I felt so lucky to be alive; other mornings I'd open my eyes and whimper with fear about what the day might bring. Those were the days I didn't get out of bed.

Though I'd lost thirty-five pounds and was lighter than I had ever been as an adult, my body felt as heavy as an anchor. It wanted to drag me down, hide me from the world and drown me.

Three months after my surgeon removed a lobe of my lung and my wound had healed, I still ached psychically. I could not seem to get back to the normal I had known before. I was depressed but did not realize it. A common side effect of cancer, the fog of depression often seeps in unnoticed. Like becoming nearsighted, it happens so slowly we sometimes fail to realize it until we run into a wall. Luckily, when I ran into my wall, I was surrounded by friends and loved ones who waited with me until the fog dissipated. They tolerated my quickly changing moods and the often odd and offensive words and actions that accompanied them.

When my dearest pal, Al, treated me to a Santana concert, which included shaking Carlos's hand backstage, I barked at her after getting lost trying to find our car in the massive parking lot. It was my first real outing since my surgery, and I had not shared with her how depressed and exhausted I felt. Having lost a lobe of my lung, my other lobes were still learning to compensate; eventually they would fill the cavity left behind by my missing sac, but for now, I became winded easily.

When we finally found the car and were driving the half hour home, Al asked me a question about my son leaving for college the next year. The thought of losing him made my heart pound with pain. I snapped back, "Can we not talk about that?" She had no idea how raw I felt, but instead of reacting with anger, as she could have, she accepted my behavior and even apologized.

A few weeks later, though I had started taking antidepressant drugs, my moods were still mercurial. My husband had taken me to a spa in Guerneville, where we had vacationed the summer before, and he pampered me all weekend with gourmet meals, slow strolls through the giant redwoods, a body massage, and later a hair treatment. The stylist's strong fingers shampooing my scalp soothed my soul, but when he started telling me of all the hair products that could smooth my frizz, he shattered my calm. Still vulnerable and hypersensitive from the trauma of cancer, I felt he was pressuring me to buy something.

> *"Don't assume you know what end of the spectrum I am on any given day. You don't have to know a thing about me or about cancer because all you have to do is ask."*
>
> —S.D., breast cancer survivor

"I just got over cancer," I said coldly, "so I really have to watch my budget." "Oh, I am so sorry!" the stylist exclaimed, and immediately left the room. A moment later he returned holding a calming green gift pack of Pevonia lotions and gels. "I have so many friends who have had AIDS and cancer. I know how hard it must be when you can't work and earn money like you used to."

The lotions and gels smelled of lemon and verbena. I have kept one of the jars, with just a smidge of lotion remaining, because it smells to me of love, and I cannot bear to part with it.

That man will never know what his small act of kindness meant to me, though I wrote him a thank-you note right away. Rather than reacting defensively, he chose to give me a gift. And it was his love, not the lotions and gels, that soothed me. Not motivated by pity, but by compassion, he forgave my bark and petted me instead.

He treated me with kid gloves, but I never noticed that he had donned them.

16.

"Hearing platitudes or what's good about cancer can trivialize my feelings."

It is better wither to be silent, or to say things of more value than science. Sooner throw a pearl at hazard than an idle or useless word.

—Pythagoras

PLATITUDES, DEFINED AS "pointless, unoriginal, or empty comments or statements made as though they were significant or helpful," can make light of what is, to some people, the heaviest of experiences: having cancer.

And, often, such statements are dead wrong.

"She's in a better place now," said a funeral attendee to a bereaved widow. "A better place would be in my arms," the widow may have wanted to reply.

"You're so lucky you caught it early," an acquaintance told Monica Powell.

"I'm thinking, 'No, lucky is when you win the lottery!' To apply that word to cancer is cruel," Monica remarked. "Some people say, 'You can use cancer to transform your life.' Well, as they say in psychotherapy, AFOG—'another f-ing opportunity for growth!'" Powell chuckled. "I transformed my life a long time ago; I already went through a horrible divorce! I already value my life! I'm already clear; it's not like I needed a kick in the butt. People saying that just ticks me off."

Platitudes, also known as clichés, are often said without much thought; they come to mind easily because they have been said before. Too often, they may come across as insincere.

To a cancer patient, who trauma has rendered raw and who is in great need of compassion and sincerity, platitudes may sting. Although what is a cliché to one person may be a "truth" to another, some common sayings seem to strike many cancer survivors as inappropriate. In this chapter, I outline some of those sayings in the hopes that you will give them a little thought before speaking them. They may not be offensive to your loved one, and if you feel compelled to offer the words anyway, why not preface them with, "I hope this doesn't trivialize what you're going through, but I'd like to offer a saying that means a lot to me."

"You could get hit by a bus"

The platitude many cancer survivors report disliking most is, "You never know how much time any of us has; you could go outside tomorrow and get hit by a bus!"

Many who've had cancer have heard at least one version of that platitude from a friend or, more often, a stranger. "I heard that maybe ten times, even by my primary care physician," said Johanna Anderson, whose lymphoma threatened to end her life of only twenty-seven years. "It was kind of like, 'Okay, so then in addition to the fact that I could die from cancer, I might also get hit by a truck!'"

Some patients say they would prefer getting flattened by a bus because then their death would be sudden and perhaps painless. Being struck by cancer is very different from accidentally walking into the path of a random vehicle; unlike getting hit by a bus, cancer grows slowly and invisibly, even deceptively. You can name the exact time a bus runs someone over, but you can never know when the cancer cells started multiplying in your body.

〜〜〜

Patti Dickerson's pet peeve is people who tell her, "This happened for a reason," or, "This happened because you can handle it." People said such things both while her husband, Louis, was suffering from multiple tumors and after the tumors killed him.

"It's sort of like a pseudo-Eastern approach, which is like there's a balance in the universe and this happened for a reason," she said, still angry years later.

"I was looking at [Rabbi Harold] Kushner's book, *When Bad Things Happen to Good People*," she continued after a few moments of silence. "The book said there is chaos in the world and things just happen. So, stop!" she snapped, making a plea to those who want to tell her Louis died for a reason.

"You've got to be strong"

Dolores Moorehead worked for the American Cancer Society for twenty years before joining the Women's Cancer Resource Center. She has heard hundreds of cancer stories, but the one that came to mind when I asked her about what to say or not say to a cancer patient was deeply personal.

"My cousin's wife had just been diagnosed with breast cancer and was going to have surgery," she began. "Her husband, my cousin, had just bought a new motorcycle. The ground was slick. He hit a tree and lay on the side of the road for hours, and he died.

"And this is where culture comes in, probably. My cousin's wife was scheduled to have her surgery that Monday, and my mother said that the best thing she did was be strong, that she went ahead and buried her husband and had her surgery and never showed any emotion."

That upset Moorehead because it didn't give her cousin's wife permission to show her feelings. "And basically that's saying that to show emotion is a sign of weakness, which I think is cultural. It's cultural that African Americans are supposed to be strong. But what a weight for her to bear to unexpectedly lose her husband when she was in the throes of needing him the most."

"It's hard to explain that it does feel different from your normal, statistical risk of being hit by a car."

—A.B., breast cancer survivor

Moorehead believes that telling anyone who has cancer to be strong is unfair. She said it, of course, takes great strength to cope with cancer, but patients need to be able to break down—to experience fear, anger, and other "negative" emotions. "People need to give you permission to do that," insisted Moorehead. "And if you're raised not to ever cry because that's a sign of weakness, then you don't have the opportunity to cry or to reach out to people."

Moorehead said we get mixed messages: On the one hand, we are encouraged to be emotional and caring, but on the other, we are expected to show strength. "I think to crumble on the floor may be seen as undignified, but I think crumbling on the floor isn't going to happen as long as you know that people around you will pick you up."

Therapist Halina Irving said if you do not crumble on the floor, healing becomes more difficult. "If we don't have to spend all our energy hiding and suppressing and repressing the fear and the despair, then there's room for the hope. If they can find someone who accepts [their fear and despair], who understands it as normal and is willing to hear it without blaming them, once they feel that and are allowed to go to the bottom, very naturally they'll start feeling better and start feeling more positive, and there will be room for hope."

> *"I loved it when friends resisted the urge to say something 'wise' to fill the silence. Sometimes the wisest words are those that remain unspoken."*
>
> —L.C., lung cancer survivor

"Everything's going to be okay" or "you'll be just fine"

"You'll be fine; I have a friend who had the same thing, and she's fine now." That's what Janice Maxwell heard from a loved one. "Nobody, including the oncologist," Janice complained, "knows if a patient will be fine. I know the statement is meant to encourage, but it trivializes the seriousness of the disease."

As Dr. Lawrence LeShan said, "Don't tell me things you don't know anything about. Don't tell me I'm going to get better; don't tell me I'm going to get worse."

Another woman, Geena, just diagnosed with breast cancer, told the story of her friend, Douglas. "Mickey Mouse is his idol. He has this little Mickey Mouse tattoo."

When she sent Douglas an email, just days after her diagnosis, he replied electronically: "Hi Geena. You'll be fine."

Geena shook her head quickly, her short black curls bouncing against her forehead. "He added a little 'blah blah blah,' you know, and then, 'Have a good day.' And I thought, 'After what I told you, how can you imagine that I'm going to have a good day for a few more days?' Now I can laugh about it, but at that point . . . "

What hurt her most about Douglas's naïve response was that it did not feel nurturing. "Douglas always says, 'I know what you're going through.' Or, 'I know how you feel.' He always gives advice. And usually he knows nothing about what I am going through—although he can be a very good listener.

"It's isolating in a way, because it says to me he really doesn't grasp what I'm going through. It doesn't make me feel closer to him. I have to back up and remember that he loves me."

As psychologist Paul Ekman said, people in pain need someone to have the emotional empathy to reverberate what they're feeling.

But some people simply cannot relate, and that's part of the reason they come up with platitudes. As noted earlier, Ekman said some people have a restrictive range of emotions and cannot deal with bad news or sick people.

Dolores Moorehead said many people just don't know how to deal with the reality of their own mortality.

"A lot of times I feel that when people say, 'You're going to be okay,' it's partly because that's what they need to hear—not so much what you need to hear. It makes them feel better, because they really don't know what to do with what's happening and how they're feeling."

> *"My neighbor said it would take me less time to get ready since I didn't have to wash my hair. That's not what I needed to hear."*
>
> —N.W., thyroid cancer survivor

"Cancer is a gift"

This platitude is related to "There's a reason the universe gave you cancer." Breast cancer survivor and activist Barbara Brenner, who leads the non-profit Breast Cancer Action, does not buy it one bit. Her response to people who remark that her cancer was a gift is, "A gift is something you would give away. To whom would you give this gift?"

"At least you get to say good-bye to your loved ones"

Personally, I appreciate the "I could get hit by a bus" remark. I see the speaker trying to put herself on the same level as me, saying in so many words, "We're mortal; we're equal. You can die, I can die."

But there's a strange irony here. Fact is, you will die, and so will I. The difference is, people with so-called "terminal" cancer have a better idea of when.

If I had a choice, I would probably choose cancer over getting hit by a bus. Although I don't want to hear how lucky I am to have had cancer (let me come to that conclusion myself, if I need to), I find that most people who have had cancer appreciate the opportunity to take a closer look at their lives.

A recent report on National Public Radio told a tale of an oncology social worker who decided to survey sixty of her peers. She asked them how they would want to die.

Oncology social workers care for people who are suffering from and sometimes dying of cancer. These providers see bones emerging out of flesh as cancer eats away fat, then muscle tissue; they see parents suffer with the knowledge that they may not see their children or grandchildren step up to middle school; they see the anguish of animal lovers who know their beloved tabby or toy fox terrier will have to go on without them; they see people of all ages who will never again take a vacation.

But oncology social workers see something else as well: terminally ill people taking the time to say good-bye to their loved ones and to put their emotional and physical houses in order.

To the researcher's surprise, almost all the respondents of her survey said they would rather die of cancer than in an auto crash or by a heart attack. Because pain is so much more effectively controlled these days, few feared physical suffering. Much more troubling to the oncology social workers was the thought of leaving things left unsaid or of not having the opportunity to say a proper good-bye.

Terminally ill people usually take advantage of the opportunity to tie up loose ends and prepare for death. Those who die suddenly can leave behind a legacy of longing or regret that lives on forever.

Jackie Kennedy said to her priest, Reverend Richard McSorley, about the assassination of her husband, "If I only had a minute to say good-bye. It was so hard not to say good-bye, not be able to say good-bye." But telling a cancer patient, "At least you get to say good-bye," trivializes that person's pain. Good-bye is good-bye.

"Cancer sucks!" (No platitude, that!)

Barbara Brenner was on vacation in Banff, Canada, in 1993 when she found a lump in her breast during her monthly self-examination. "I figured it was a cyst," she said, offhandedly. "When I got home I called my doctor."

Brenner had breast cancer. She took a leave of absence from her law firm, and in the midst of treatment she realized she wanted to work in women's health. Within two years, she had become executive director of Breast Cancer Action.

"I'm very privileged, very privileged to be able to do this. We're at a critical point in trying to figure this stuff out, and if we don't figure it out soon, everybody is going to have breast cancer."

Brenner says women now have a one in seven chance of developing breast cancer during their lifetime. Her organization is dedicated to ending the epidemic by finding the causes and eliminating them, finding a true cure with treatments that don't kill people or cause other diseases, and advocating for universal access to quality health care.

"When someone says, 'It's God's will,' I feel like it's a hopeless situation. And why would God want me to suffer like this?"

—I.N., pancreatic cancer survivor

Although Breast Cancer Action is a political and activist organization, it also provides support and information to newly diagnosed women. It provides a flyer, "What to Do When Someone You Know Has Been Diagnosed with Breast Cancer."

I saw the flyer when I attended the organization's annual Town Hall meeting as an editor for *Bay Area Business Woman.* I was impressed with the advice it listed: listen to her; offer a shoulder to cry on; don't say what you would do in her situation; give advice only when asked; offer to accompany her to doctor appointments; offer to drive her to and from treatments; organize family and friends to help with household needs such as babysitting, housecleaning, and food preparation; get support for yourself; and join Breast Cancer Action!

But I was even more impressed with the big white-and-red buttons and stickers piled on the table by the entrance door in the reception area that read: "Cancer Sucks."

When I heard my son say "sucks" for the first time when he was sixteen, I was offended. Normally, I find that word vulgar. But when paired with "cancer," it sounds perfectly appropriate. Although "suck" may be a crude word, cancer is a crude, obscene, vulgar disease, and why not call a spade a spade? It's hard to understand cancer's obscenity unless you have experienced it in your own body or through a loved one.

I thought printing "Cancer Sucks" on a button was a brilliant way to get the word out—especially to youth—about Breast Cancer Action and the horror of the disease.

Brenner explained the slogan's genesis. A woman on the Breast Cancer Action board, Lucy Sherack, had a recurrence of breast cancer and was told she didn't have a lot of time left to live. "She was very upset and she said, 'I've developed this button that says, "Cancer Sucks," and we've got to use it.' And then Lucy died."

Breast Cancer Action not only used her idea, they turned it into a banner statement. "We made a big deal about the button, largely because it was important from that personal connection to this really wonderful woman who left two teenaged children and a devoted husband when she died, and because it was important for the public to begin to understand that whatever it looks like is going on in [cancer research], 'progress' is being covered up by the failure to tell the truth about what is going on.

"I have a Cancer Sucks button on almost every outer piece of clothing I own," Brenner said, "and people see them and they say, 'Wow!' People resonate with them. It starts conversations. People say, 'Yeah, cancer does suck.' Because it does; it's a terrible disease."

Cancer is also a disease that inspires soul searching and questions that may never be answered. Before you ask what seems to some the most logical question, "Why did my friend or loved one get cancer?," please read on.

17.

"I don't know why I got cancer, and I don't want to know your theory."

A man thinks that by mouthing hard words he understands hard things.

—Herman Melville

I STARTED SMOKING CIGARETTES because I thought it was cool. It was right before the U.S. Surgeon General declared "Smoking may be hazardous to your health," but knowing that would not have stopped me. I was a teenager, and although I wanted to look older, I never gave a thought to *growing* older than my midtwenties, when I imagined I would be married to Lanny and have a gaggle of kids.

Lanny was my first official boyfriend. After ceremoniously giving me the silver I.D. bracelet that bore his real name, Jesse Landis, he taught me how to breathe cigarette smoke into my lungs while we picnicked in Shaw Park on humid summer days, as teens and children swam gleefully in the pool complex a couple of hundred yards away. It was thrilling to show off my glamour, my sophistication, my "cool."

I quit in the mid-1980s, long after cigarettes had been upgraded from "hazardous" to "dangerous," and after many previous attempts. Quitting was more difficult than anything I had ever done, but I was in my late twenties and had not only started believing in my mortality but also had come to believe that tobacco companies exploited youth. I abhorred the impact of secondhand smoke and the horror of addiction.

Having been overexposed to breast cancer through my personal experiences—two very dear first cousins had suffered from it, and I had worked on two documentaries about it—I thought that that would be the kind of crab to pinch me. So when I was diagnosed with lung cancer almost twenty years after I had quit smoking, I was shocked. But not nearly as shocked as people who had never known me as a smoker.

"But you're not a smoker!" they would exclaim.

"I quit almost twenty years ago," I'd answer defensively, feeling guilty that I was to blame for the disease that might kill me. It added the proverbial insult to injury. Not only had I caused my own cancer, I could have prevented it, and now I would be judged for it.

I had many secret theories (as most cancer patients do) about why I had gotten cancer, and most did not have anything to do with smoking. They had more to do with transgressions dating back to my second boyfriend, whose heart I broke. Then there was the workaholism of which so many had accused me, and so on.

But enough about my secret theories. I know now that they were ridiculous. I got cancer partly because I smoked—though a new study from Duke University shows that fifteen years after quitting smoking, most Americans can expect to live as long as those who never smoked. In addition, plenty of people smoke longer and more than I did and never get lung cancer, and way too many people—especially women—who never smoked suffer from the disease.

For instance, Jimmie Holland's daughter-in-law. When I interviewed Dr. Holland, the legendary psychiatrist and founder of the field of psychoon-cology, she told me her son's wife was dying of lung cancer. Just thirty-seven years old, she seemed to have run out of treatment options.

I asked Dr. Holland whether people asked her daughter-in-law if she smoked.

"You know, I don't know," replied Dr. Holland, puzzled. "But I find myself saying that she never smoked, which is kind of interesting; why I have to say that is interesting."

Her daughter-in-law not only was a nonsmoker but had no other risk factors.

"Why did she get it?" asked Dr. Holland. "Was it in her family? No, it's not in her family. People want to establish a cause, particularly when it's a young person and it's unexpected. If you can attribute a cause then you can say, 'It won't happen to me, I don't smoke so I'm safe'—it's a sort of 'you and not me' situation. If we can figure out why it happened, well, then it won't happen to me."

Cancer happened to Jamie Danforth; he was afflicted with a rare form, cancer of the tonsils.

"I didn't blame myself; I hadn't had a drink for twenty years or been much of a smoker," he explained.

Because the disease is so uncommon, Jamie says, people didn't say much about it. And as one protective of his privacy, he did not feel comfortable talking about it. But there was one person in his life with whom he did discuss the disease: his girlfriend.

"She was a singer. And she said that because I didn't use my voice, my voice was being taken away from me," Jamie explained matter-of-factly. "I never had a great voice, but now I was taken a notch down. She meant this in an expressive way, not just literally, like, 'You need to speak up for yourself, here I am.'

"I think because she was a singer, saying that was her protection, like, 'This is why it won't happen to me.' I was sitting next to her, and I just said, 'Oh,' but by the end of her saying that, she knew she was on thin ice."

Why me? Why *not* me?

Diana Delaney understands grief and loss, and the awkwardness of talking about it to people who haven't been through it. At twenty-seven, with an interest in social work, she did an internship at a children's grief support group program. Although she wanted to be a social worker, she did not get into the social work school of her choice; instead, years later, she entered a different but similar field.

"I'm in nursing school, and I'm interested in oncology and hospice," she explained, sitting down in my sunny office on a ninety-degree August day. "Everyone wants to be a labor-delivery nurse because it's 'happy' nursing. But within nursing it makes sense to me to make a difference in the less fun parts. Nursing is not so different from grief work and social work. I felt that in some way I could combine my previous experiences and inclinations with the huge thing that happened in my life."

The huge thing that happened in Diana's life was the stuff of a movie script, the kind of tragic story that begs for some meaningful explanation.

Like a movie star, Diana's beauty was stunning; with not a dab of makeup, her faintly freckled dark skin radiated health and inner warmth. Her light brown hair had straw-colored streaks and hung over her shoulders, falling forward as she leaned over to tell her tale.

"A few people act as if you might be contagious or had done something to deserve the disease. Now, that really hurt, I suppose because of the little nagging voice inside that's saying the same thing."

—D.A., Hodgkins survivor

I learned that her physical beauty was matched by her formidable inner spirit. She told me a story that she had not shared for a very long time, a story that's difficult for her to tell, so readers of this book might keep others from experiencing the kind of pain inflicted on and her husband, Baruch.

"Baruch's a California boy by way of Argentina," Diana laughed. "Baruch is actually a Hebrew name which means 'blessed'— and he was a blessing to me.

"It's kind of like a Jewish epic story," she continued. "His grandparents were Holocaust survivors from Poland who fled to Argentina after the war. Baruch was born there in 1971 and then moved to Los Angeles with his parents, who planned to move to Israel. But they never made it."

Baruch's mother was a pediatrician, Diana said, and in a way Baruch became his mother's patient. When he was twenty-two, he was diagnosed with osteoblastoma, which appeared as tumors on his spine. By the time he and Diana met six years later, he would have had eight spinal surgeries. In between the operations, Diana said Baruch had led an active life like other men his age.

"He had become a teacher and had traveled and had a love life and had friends and went to rock concerts and all this stuff. But there was this ongoing medical battle."

They met through friends a few years before they started dating; both had been seeing someone else at the time, so they didn't act on their mutual attraction. But when Baruch was single again and heard Diana was too, he caller her for a date.

"One thing led to another, and we moved in together three months later," Diana smiled. She paused; the curve of her mouth dropped. "Three months later, he had a ninth surgery. It was a 'normal' recovery in Baruch's life, in the sense that he would go, get this harrowing surgery, be in the hospital for a week, return to Los Angeles for four or five weeks to recover, and then resume his life, which he had done in the years before I met him. So this was kind of routine for him.

"He lived in chronic pain. And he kind of kept marching on, like it was all very normal—even though in retrospect it was so insane."

What made it less insane was his mother's medical sophistication. "It was other people's job to worry about his medical treatment. And so he just knew that everything was going to be okay. I think when you're a grown-up the enormity of it hits you in a different way." Diana said Baruch was more like a child. "It was just a part of his psyche to get back up and go on."

"Two different acquaintances suggested that I had brought on my own cancer through negative thoughts! Even though I didn't believe it for a second, it outraged me that someone else believed it."

—F.P., sarcoma survivor

Diana and Baruch went on to the next natural step for two young people in love: They set a date to be married. A few months after their engagement, another tumor appeared.

"The indication that the tumor had recurred was always increased pain. And so in the fall of 2000, his pain level kept climbing, and it got to a place where we couldn't be out for more than two hours before he would need to get home and ice his back. And he became more weak and less mobile."

Together, Diana and Baruch went to Baltimore so he could get another operation. "At that point, he'd been through a major course of radiation and had ten spinal surgeries and major reconstruction. He was just thirty years old, and your body can only take so much. When he woke up from that surgery, he couldn't feel or move his legs."

After several more weeks in Baltimore, he returned home, in a wheelchair, and experienced more medical complications. Again, he went to the hospital.

"He contracted meningitis," Diana said, looking deeply into my eyes. "And then August of 2001 the tumor recurred, and we were right back to square one and he hadn't even begun to heal from the prior hospitalizations. Everything had spun out of control until it just got worse and worse and worse and then . . .

"I don't know exactly what I'm supposed to be talking about," she said, crying.

I shared her tears, and share them again as I recall our conversation. Although she said she had told the story a million times, she had not told it for many months and had not told it in such a focused way.

They married three weeks before he died, knowing that he was dying. They had postponed the October wedding until June, not knowing that his disease was terminal. But when he developed an unstoppable infection, they knew he was going to die. He chose to discontinue treatment.

"He wanted so much to know that people accepted that choice; he had really checked in with his inner self, with the cosmos, and said he needed people to understand and respect that."

"Did they?" I asked.

"Those people closest to him did, but some people in our community just couldn't imagine in a time of medical miracles that we couldn't fix it; it was just unfathomable to them."

What Diana found difficult to accept was the number of people who speculated to her about why all of this was happening to her and Baruch.

"At first they did that when Baruch was sick. If I were going through that I'd be angry and bitter, but instead his heart just got bigger and bigger. He got life's priorities straight and was very easy with himself and non-judgmental."

Diana said sometimes people would say things meant to be complimentary, but they hurt her deeply. "They'd be like, 'Baruch is so special, so amazing; Baruch's so strong; you're so strong. This happened because you guys can handle it.' That kind of thing. It's an attempt to give you credit for handling things well, but sometimes I felt like, 'Let me get this straight: If our relationship weren't so strong and beautiful he wouldn't have gotten sick?'"

ΞΞΞ

Diana said such well-meaning comments continued after Baruch died. "That we can glean knowledge or create meaning is not the reason [bad things] happen. Being able to understand, to pour out the loss of what has happened is a different experience from why it happened."

Most people who have experienced loss can understand what Diana was talking about. Why do bad things happen to good people? Is it God's will? Are those who smoke immoral or weak? What about workaholics who give more to their jobs than their families?

"I was brought up in the Catholic faith," said Jill Jordan, who used to work for an AIDS food bank, "and to say that God would put down someone because of a lifestyle is just ridiculous." Jill said that since she worked at the food bank, many people assumed she had AIDS and looked down on her. "The rudeness of people—how could you blame someone for having it? You see the very positive and very negative sides of people."

Jill soon came to be judged for a disease she did have. Diagnosed with late-stage lung cancer, she was asked frequently whether and how much she smoked. "Lung cancer is one of the most degrading cancers, and it doesn't matter whether you smoked. You have it. I get offended by that. I smoked a long time ago. I agree people should stop smoking. And I did, twelve years ago. But I had had cancer for at least ten years when they diagnosed it."

Beyond "why?"

I do not know how long I had cancer before it was diagnosed. I showed no symptoms; the very small tumor was discovered by mistake—or by Providence—when I got a CT scan of my abdomen. The tumor must have started growing long after I quit smoking, but perhaps the genetic damage was done during my years as a smoker. What made my tumor form? Was it my workaholism? Was it breathing polluted air?

Who knows? What matters now is that I live on. As does Jill. You can help people like us continue living and living happily by not trying to figure out why we got cancer. We may have already searched our minds and souls for the answer.

As therapists Pat Fobair, Marty Marder, and Sheila Slattery wrote in "Resilience, a Patients Perspective," "We don't blame our pets when they get cancer. Why do we blame ourselves?"

"You can't help but wonder, 'Why did this thing happen?'" said Dr. Holland. "Why did the earthquake hit my house and not another one? Why did the disease hit my grandson? Why, why, why, why, why? There isn't any answer, and if you go there, it doesn't lead you anywhere good."

You can help us live by leading us to the good places—and by staying there with us.

18.

"I need you to understand if I don't return your call or want to see you."

Selfishness is not living as one wishes to live, it is asking others to live as one wishes to live.

—Oscar Wilde

NANA—MY FATHER'S MOTHER, Sophie Dawidoff—was an American-born German with smooth skin the color of pink clouds at sunset. After World War I, she married a Russian immigrant, Samuel Krazilchekov (translated to "Crasilneck" at Ellis Island) and committed herself to raising her family and providing her children with what she was deprived of as a child—the freedom to become whatever they dreamed.

Nana did a wonderful job raising my dad (who was apparently a hellion on wheels as a tyke) and his sister, Dorothy. For them, Nana cooked, cleaned, and simply stayed home. She did leave her house a couple of days a week, though; one to play mah-jongg, the other to volunteer at "the home," a nursing home.

I wish I had listened to her more carefully when she conveyed stories about all her friends there. As a normal self-centered teenager, I saw her not as a human being, but as Nana the nurturer, Nana the rescuer, Nana the best angel food cake–maker on earth.

I do remember the way her face used to relax into a proud smile when she told me about the bounty of birthday cards she received each year from her friends at the home.

Later in my life, when I entered my twenties and thirties, the number of envelopes in my mailbox on the day of my birth came to signify how much I was loved. Fortunately, I had two sets of grandparents and two sets of aunts and uncles who never forgot to send a greeting card (and usually a check). But my favorite card always came from Rosie, our cleaning lady.

Rosie had shiny dark brown skin and a maternal aroma of fried eggs and Jergen's lotion that stayed in our kitchen for hours after she went home. When I was a child, she would hand me an envelope that contained a card on my birthday, sometimes dusted with glitter, signed with two of the only words she knew how to read or write: "Love, Rosie." The card would always contain a brand new dollar bill or two, which, as I grew older, meant more to me than gifts that were exponentially more expensive.

> *"I had a friend who kept calling and leaving messages asking how I was doing and why I hadn't called back. When I finally did, he asked if he could call me later!"*
>
> —T.R., prostate cancer survivor

As my aunts and uncles passed away (they all died too young), my yearly card collection dwindled to a pile of three or four. Sometimes friends or cousins would send cards. When they did not, I would feel a little tinge of pain though I always trusted their love. It was Nana's legacy that led me to invest so much emotional stock in the U.S. Postal Service. (Now I delight in e-cards!)

Delightful Surprises

Two days after I was diagnosed with cancer, I sent out a mass email to some three hundred friends and colleagues. Never one to ask for help, suddenly I was enlisting the support of folks I barely knew. I was certain I was going to need every bit of good will I could harness.

In my email alert I asked people to pray for me or keep me in their thoughts. Within a matter of minutes, it was as if the top of a water hydrant had burst open. Love, sweet words, and gifts rushed forth, arriving via cyberspace, airspace, freeway, and telephone line. Even my corporate and government clients left voice mails in tones I'd never before heard from them; two even said, in all earnestness, "I love you."

It was the other kind of mail that shocked me the most. Greeting cards arrived like spring rains. Sometimes there would be a little shower, other times my mailbox would be deluged, which would make my heart overflow with feelings impossible to describe.

Then there were the gifts. Fragrant candles and incense; Hello Kitty pens and pads; novels; books about healing, nutrition, and meditation; books pregnant with words of wisdom, such as *Words on Calm*; cassette tapes and CDs; stationery; and on and on.

I'm not writing this to brag; almost every cancer patient I have met has received an outpouring like the one I experienced. It's one of the miracles of illness: Love bursts through like seedlings whose seeds you never knew were planted.

What was difficult for me, however, was maintaining the back-and-forth flow of information I desired. Although I wanted to respond to everyone's gifts and questions about my health and treatment, I was so busy driving from doctor to doctor, spending time with family who had traveled halfway across the country for me, and meditating (to keep my head from exploding), that I couldn't return all the telephone calls and emails I got. I did send out a couple of mass emails, but it felt too impersonal, and even though I thought my friends would understand, I felt guilty about not taking more time to respond personally. The problem was, I didn't *have* the time; I was so busy, as therapist Halina Irving said, "running from the tiger in the woods," I could not stop for fear of losing my very life.

Rabbi Natan Fenner of Bay Area Jewish Healing Center, whose wife had recently undergone treatment for breast cancer, told me about a website called CaringBridge (www.caringbridge.org). The site enabled visitors to access a special web page to read an update on her health; you could also send an email message of any length, if you wanted.

I told my teenaged son, Brett, about the site, and before I knew it, he was creating a web page just for me.

Friday, July 12, 2002 at 08:39 p.m. (CDT)

This page has just been created. Please check back for additional updates. Any information about Lori's surgery, meetings, care, etc., will be posted in journal entries.

The next entry read:

Saturday, July 20, 2002 at 11:37 p.m. (CDT)

Lori will be going into surgery this Monday morning at Kaiser in Oakland. The surgery will start at about 8:00 in the morning, and (knock on wood) be over at about 11:00. (So any good vibes/prayers would be well received around that time). I will post something in the late afternoon on this website, letting everyone know how things went. After that, Lori will spend a few days in ICU, and about a week after the surgery will be home to recover.

I will be posting any new information on this website, as well as perhaps posting requests for help, should the need arise. We probably won't be sending out any more mass emails after Monday. Lori wanted me to thank all of you for all of your love and support, and just wanted to ask you to forgive her if she doesn't respond in a timely fashion to any emails or phone calls. You can also post things in the guest book on this web page, and I will print them out and give them to Lori when she is feeling well enough to read them, but Lori didn't want me to discourage you from sending her emails as well. Thank you all.

—Brett

Free and available for anyone who has an illness, CaringBridge web pages are easy to set up and administer. The value of mine was immeasurable; it created a conduit for love and humor. (My brother, Ron, wrote, "Lori, now you be nice to the hospital staff! You don't want to be any trouble! I wish Suzy and I and all the kids could have been there today, but they probably wouldn't have let me do any of the surgery anyway. . . . Seriously, take it easy and don't try to do too much too fast. We all love you. Your Bro")

During those two months, I received more than one hundred Caring-Bridge messages from people, some I didn't even know, in addition to the hundreds of emails friends and colleagues sent. Everyone sounded so selfless; for once, it was all about me. It was like my birthday, and it was, in fact, a birth-day of sorts. I had survived the surgery, which I had feared as if it were an execution, certainly not a blessing (which it was).

All told, the support—the calls, emails, website messages, and greeting cards—created an ocean on which I felt I could float forever.

A few weeks after surgery, when my father came for another visit, he helped me hang seven thin rows of wrapping paper ribbons of satin white, pale pink, and lime green across the wall next to my bed. Pulled tight, we placed all the get-well cards over them. There were so many, we had to overlap them. Several friends sent multiple greetings, some funny, some elegantly simple, all simply beautiful. Some cards dropped sparkles like angel dust onto the floor; some burst forth with colorful bouquets or single calla lily blooms; some showed puppy eyes; one cartoon greeting revealed the backside of an old man in a hospital gown.

Two years after my diagnosis, the cards remained on my wall. I have reread them several times. I keep thinking I should take them down. "It's time to move on," my inner voice suggests gently. But I cannot seem to let even one go: I have even kept the two-by-four-inch cards that accompanied the flowers and plants.

> *"One friend did not understand when I told her that I didn't want any phone calls, that I needed time to go inside myself to work through the pain. She was offended. I was angry that she didn't value my feelings."*
>
> —S.W., breast cancer survivor

Weeks after my surgery, I tried to return twofold as much love as all the friends, loved ones, and strangers had put into those cards. Creating a ritual of penning thank-you notes allowed love to circulate through my embattled body and soul and then come back out. It made me all the stronger. Basically, it helped me live. But often I was too tired to return the phone calls and could not always accept visitors, especially while I was in the midst of treatment and recovery.

Sometimes I felt guilty when a friend would ask when she could come over and give me a hug. How could I deny someone the opportunity to share their love, especially when I needed to receive it as much as they needed to give it?

What I realize now is that, when I feel the urge to visit a friend who has cancer, I can leave a voicemail, letting them off the hook. I can preface my message with, "No need to call me back," or, "If you're up to it, I'd love to visit, but otherwise, just know I love you."

Elizabeth's story

She walked like a dancer or Carmen Miranda balancing a basket of apples, coconuts, and bananas atop her head. Graceful, muscular, and slim, but not rib-thin, her body seemed almost perfect. In the step aerobics classes she taught, she wore black leotards and a white Lycra sleeveless top that revealed her tan and miraculously flat belly. How old was she? Mid-forties? Hard to tell: She had the energy of a teen and the enthusiasm and openness of a child.

I walked into her class for the first time, shy and scared. Overweight and frumpy in the extra large black T-shirt that hid my rear, I set up my teal plastic platform in the very back of the mirrored room. This was Advanced Step, and I had been "stepping" only about three months. Those in the front rows were fit; there could not have been more than ten pounds of fat between the four of them.

Elizabeth McWilliams walked like a dancer because she was one. Her creatively choreographed step routines, which changed weekly, challenged her students to move quickly and unconsciously. You almost had to let your body take over; if you let your mind anticipate your moves, you'd get lost.

I credit Elizabeth with helping me live. Years before my cancer diagnosis, during a bout with depression that lasted more than a year, I often felt on the brink of self-destruction, not through suicide, but via disease. My immune system was on overload, and I feared I would fall prey to the disease that had killed my best friend and my cousin. Elizabeth's step routines helped me drop thirty pounds, lower my cholesterol and stress levels, and ratchet up my self-esteem.

"I loved having people leave 'I'm thinking about you messages' and not expecting me to call them back."

—T.S., breast cancer survivor

It turns out I had been growing a tumor anyway, probably for at least a decade. Who knows why. Was it fed by my depression? Probably not. But I know that the thrice-weekly classes with Elizabeth helped me perspire and release fluids, which, like crying, felt cathartic.

When I got cancer, I stopped attending Elizabeth's classes. After a while, I went to the club to put my membership on hold—I knew it would take months to be able to strenuously work out again—and I ran into her.

"I have missed you so much!" I almost shouted. "I hope you didn't think I stopped coming because of you. It's actually that I have cancer, and I've been overwhelmed with doctor's appointments."

She cocked her head a little and lowered her chin. "That's shitty!" she said, a crease forming between her blue eyes.

Had those words really come out of that sweet mouth with the innocent smile?

I was thrilled—not to hear a curse word—but to know that Elizabeth cared enough about me to sympathize so intensely. She was not judging me, only the cancer that threatened my life.

"How are you doing with it?" she asked, head still tilted slightly, and I blathered on about the terror, the insecurity, the confusion I felt. She looked at me lovingly, but not condescendingly; she listened and nodded and took my hand.

222

I did not think there was anything that could disappoint me more than having to give up the step class I had been attending faithfully for half a decade. Once I had recovered from my surgery—I'd given myself a good six months—I returned to the club, only to find that Elizabeth would soon be leaving. An ankle injury she had sustained as a dancer had been worsening, and she could no longer teach. I videotaped her last class and interviewed her students, some of whom must have climbed a thousand miles of steps with her during the last fifteen years. Everyone had signed an oversize greeting card for her before class; afterward, I made a dub of the tape and mailed it with the card, stamped with all the love I had.

I didn't hear from her that summer, and I assumed that, as a mother of two boys, aged seven and nine, she was more overwhelmed than I. Neglecting to acknowledge a gift for a while is perfectly understandable when you're raising children—especially when they're out of school—so I didn't give it a thought. But when I got a letter from her the next fall, everything made sense—in the most disturbing way possible.

"I'm so sorry I never wrote to you, I meant to, a hundred times," she wrote in penmanship as delicate as her cheekbones. "But I was diagnosed with breast cancer, and it has been a whirlwind. You know."

Shit! I thought, then shouted. "Shit!" I immediately picked up the phone to call her.

"Elizabeth, that's shitty!" I said when she answered.

"Well, you know what it's like."

"What can I do? What can I bring you?"

"How about yourself?" she asked.

⧉⧉⧉

I was not surprised at all to find family photos on Elizabeth's walls that beamed smiles like halogen; the walnut built-ins fit perfectly with her character; and the beautiful antique furniture upholstered in deep burgundies and forest greens matched her warmth and humility.

"Let's go sit by the pool," she said.

I felt like a teacher's pet and delighted in the attention. In my mind she was one of those undiscovered luminaries, content to light its own nearby skies without acclaim. As Elizabeth and I learned more about one another, I told her about this book.

"Oh, do I have a story for you!" she laughed, as so many other cancer survivors had. Cancer tales are like war stories; though you may be able to laugh afterward, living through them can be torturous.

"I have this friend in the Northwest, Adrienne," she began. "She's brilliant. Huge heart," she continued. "We've been friends since high school.

"So I'm diagnosed with cancer, and my husband and I send an email out to all our friends to let them know. Then we start with all the tests, X-rays, you know the drill." I knew it too well.

"So Adrienne calls me and leaves me a message on our phone machine, saying she hopes I'm okay and I should call her," Elizabeth continued. "I'm so overwhelmed with what's happening to me and what's going to happen to me, and with my sons and family, that at the end of the day I'm so exhausted I can't remember which toothbrush is mine." She shook her head. I leaned forward, thinking I knew what was coming.

"Don't wait for the person with cancer to call or ask for help. YOU should call and initiate a visit, a movie, dinner. Lend an ear."

—E.K., leukemia survivor

"So then Adrienne calls again a couple of days later. I don't even remember her calling before, you know?" Elizabeth said, not stopping to hear my answer. "This time she leaves me a different kind of message: She says to me, 'Hey, Elizabeth, what's going on? Why aren't you calling me back? I'm worried. Give me a call. I need to hear how you're doing!'

"I meant to call Adrienne back that night," Elizabeth explained, "but my nine-year-old comes home with poison oak."

She rolled her eyes. "So the next day Adrienne calls again, and she leaves another message on my machine. She says, 'Elizabeth, my husband says I'm just being a selfish bitch, but I really need you to call me!'"

Trying not to laugh, I blurted, "She *was* being a selfish bitch! This is not supposed to be about her," I added, exasperated. "When you have cancer, it's supposed to be about *you*!"

Elizabeth and I laughed and enjoyed the dimming light in the late afternoon sky. After our visit, we lost touch with one another for a few months, as she endured chemotherapy with the support of her family, friends, and fans. I sent her a greeting card, sealed with a kiss and a prayer.

19.
"I want my caregiver to take good care of herself or himself."

Please don't tell me to relax—
it's only my tension that's holding me together.

—Ashleigh Brilliant

THERE WAS A TIME WHEN I had only myself to take care of. And I wasn't doing a very good job of it. Producing prime-time television documentaries for an NBC station—sometimes several in one year—I had little time for anything else. Although the topics were depressing, I told myself they were hopeful in that they offered solutions to grave social injustices, such as people with mental illness wandering the streets, bleeding tears, and spewing invectives like bile; teen moms needing parents but instead bearing babies; children tolerating beatings by their parents and offering enduring love to their abusers.

Ultimately, I realized what I needed was to *practice* love rather than expect to receive it myself. "You love your documentary subjects more than you love me," a boyfriend complained. He was right. So I broke up with him and got a dog.

"I am a good dog," read the headline in the *Oregonian* newspaper column. Griffin, a small German shepherd mix, had been dumped in a city park with a note attached to his collar explaining that, although he was a good dog, "my owners couldn't take care of me, so they left it up to me to find a home." The letter, written in pencil on lined notebook paper, was signed, "A broken home, a broken heart."

I tracked down the couple, Bonnie and Bruce, who had found Griffin. As sweet as Superman's foster parents, they served me champagne on Christmas Day and awarded me full custody of the frisky young pooch. Adopting Griffin was one of the best things I ever did for myself.

During my teens, my heart had been broken by divorce and abandonment (at the same time my father left my mother, my first boyfriend left me), so I had kept my ticker tightly stitched. But when I saw Griffin, my heart opened like the Red Sea, and my love rushed through like throngs of Israelites toward freedom. When I stroked Griffin's lustrous rabbit-soft coat and smelled his head, sweet as a puppy's, I melted.

I loved having to rise early each morning to walk Griffin. Even in the pouring Portland rains, he could discern the invisible scent of other neighborhood dogs and would lift his leg every ten feet or so to mark his boundary. I loved escaping at lunchtime whenever possible to drive the five miles home for a quick ball game with Griffin, and I couldn't wait to return home from work to feed him.

Years later, when I moved to the San Francisco Bay Area for a job as senior producer at a communications firm, I traveled frequently to the East Coast. My workdays that spring often lasted as long as the day's light, so I would awaken predawn to take Griffin to a thickly forested park high in the Oakland hills, where I would scribble in my journal as the sun rose while he savored the scent of deer and squirrels.

Griffin may have saved my life. I was miserable in the job that had taken me away from my best friends and my beloved Oregon family. Though I was hired to produce documentaries, I was being told who to interview for the company's film about breast cancer. Although I was as interested in cause, cure, and prevention, I was directed to focus only on treatment. Even more disturbing, I was indirectly directed by one of the funders, the pharmaceutical company that manufactured a leading breast cancer drug, to focus on its remedy. I considered myself a journalist,

"One of my wife's friends bought her a massage while I was in treatment. That made me feel so much better than if the friend had bought one for me!"

—D.D., melanoma survivor

and an ethical one, and being told how to spin or slant my stories went against everything I believed in.

Around the same time, my cousin Barbara told me about a book, *Grace and Grit,* which recounted the story of a woman, Treya Killam Wilber, living with and dying from breast cancer. I read it slowly so I could digest it fully. Written by her husband, Ken Wilber, a highly respected philosopher and author, it comprised excerpts from Treya's journals interspersed with his narrative. Deep and difficult, but bursting with as much love as pain, the book chronicled Treya's treatment, growth, and death, leaving a legacy as powerful as any I had known.

Toward the end of the summer, as I was nearing the end of *Grace and Grit* and working twelve-hour days, Griffin began gnawing on the door of the room that confined him during the day. (The woman from whom I rented asked that I keep him in my bedroom.) It struck me as unfair, unhealthy, and unkind to continue living this way—for Griffin and for me.

That, and the pressure from the documentary sponsors, pushed me to plan my escape. I saved my dollars like the nuts the squirrels outside were gathering for autumn, and three months later, on a September morning over breakfast in an elegant Washington, D.C., restaurant, I told the company president, "I'm sorry, but I can't do this anymore." She offered some paid time off to treat what she thought was burnout, but I refused.

I moved into a less expensive home, and just a few weeks later, I accompanied my cousin Barbara and her husband, Eddie, to a hospital to have a lump in her breast biopsied.

"I have cancer," she mouthed flatly, emerging in a wheelchair after the procedure, eyes wide in a face as gray-blue as the fluorescent lights above.

That night, we huddled around Barbara's kitchen table with our dear friend Dick, sharing wine and fear and grief and love. Because I had broken out of the prison of my work, I was able to offer my time and support to Barbara in a way that otherwise would have been impossible.

"When I had cancer, one of my friends would take my husband out for spicy meals. Keeping him healthy and happy was a definite key to success."

—A.S., cervical cancer survivor

Because I had taken care of myself, I was able to take care of Barbara. And I was able to take care of Griffin, who had taught me how to love again.

Because I had read *Grace and Grit,* I understood love and cancer in a whole new way. I had no idea that I would encounter Ken and Treya almost a decade later, under entirely different circumstances.

When the student is ready, the teacher will appear

I had just begun researching this book and was poring through the tall putty-colored metal file drawers at the Women's Cancer Resource Center, a nonprofit organization that offers support to women with cancer. I lifted out a large folder labeled "Caregivers" and leafed through the brochures, articles, and pamphlets for friends and loved ones of cancer patients. One of the articles jogged my memory and shouted for my attention: "What Kind of Help Really Helps?" by Treya Killam Wilber. I didn't recognize it at the time, but the essay had been excerpted from *Grace and Grit.*

It both encouraged and discouraged me. It contained almost everything I wanted to share in my book. And it was beautifully written—clear, descriptive, brimming with human interest stories, compassion, and humor. Her blunt descriptions of what helped and hurt cut straight to the heart, but gently. She addressed the issue of giving advice to people with cancer.

"At times," she wrote, "especially when decisions about treatment options loom ahead of them, people want information. They may want me to tell them about alternatives or help them research conventional therapies. Once they've chosen their treatment plan, however, they usually don't need more information, even though it may be the easiest and least threatening thing for me to give. Now they need support. They don't need to hear about the dangers of the radiation or chemotherapy or the Mexican clinic they've chosen, a choice usually made with great difficulty after long deliberation. My coming to them at this point with new suggestions about healers or techniques or therapies might only throw them back into confusion, might make them feel I doubt the path they've chosen and thus fuel their own doubts."

Treya's writing was so clear and on-target that I questioned my own purpose, my own talent, my own foray into book writing. But a careful rereading of the chapter reminded me of why I had undertaken this project. People ask questions that are intended to help, but like the query, "Did you smoke?" they can conjure guilt.

Treya continued, "If someone asks me a question like, 'Why did you choose to give yourself cancer?' it often feels like they're coming from a righteous place, a place of separation where they are well and I am sick. . . . 'Why' questions usually lead to feelings of guilt and self-blame, to regrets about the past . . . to fierce resolutions about the future that may be difficult to keep and only lead to guilt when broken. . . .

"I wanted a friend or two of my spouse's to take him out for a drink, as I knew that he needed support—especially the second time around."

—R.C., bilateral breast cancer survivor

"People sensitive to the complexity of the situation might ask a more helpful question, something like, 'How are you choosing to use this cancer?' For me, this question is exciting; it helps me look at what I can do now, helps me feel empowered and supported and challenged in a positive way. . . . In our Judeo-Christian culture, with its pervasive emphasis on sin and guilt, illness is too easily seen as punishment for wrongdoing. I prefer a more Buddhist approach where everything that happens is taken as an opportunity to increase compassion, to serve others."

I realized that my cancer had given me the opportunity to share Treya Killam Wilber's words with perhaps a new audience, and to share my own stories and mirror those of others with the goal of providing comfort and love in the midst of great suffering.

What I didn't realize was that I would also be given the opportunity to share her husband's wisdom.

It was at a "Cancer as a Turning Point" conference in San Rafael, California, that I rediscovered Ken Wilber in an article he had written for the *Journal of Transpersonal Psychology*. A stack of the reprinted eighteen-page piece, piled a foot high on one of the tables amidst other cancer paraphernalia, caught my eye. Though printed simply in fourteen-point black font on white paper, "On Being a Support Person" jumped out from among the brightly colored flyers, booklets, and pamphlets that surrounded it. The exhibition space was crowded with men and women who, in spite of balding from chemotherapy, were emboldened by the force of shared resilience.

I stopped to grab the reprint, then moved slowly on toward the door to find a place to read, undisturbed, outside.

The article began: "For almost five years now my wife, Treya, has been battling cancer and for five years I have been serving—sometimes well, sometimes not—as primary support person for her."

What followed was the "grit" I'd come to love in *Grace and Grit*. It told the honest truth, recalling the strength of a sometimes ugly and even repulsive reality. Wilber wrote about the difficulties of caregiving—something every caregiver and every ill person should read. (And I don't use the word "should" lightly.)

Mr. Wilber has kindly granted me permission to reprint parts of his article. A few of my favorite excerpts follow. For a reprint of the complete article, please see the resources section in the back of this book.

"As far as support people go, a particularly insidious problem begins to set in after about two or three months of caregiving. It is, after all, comparatively easy to deal with the outer, physical and obvious aspects of caregiving. You rearrange your work schedule; you get used to cooking, washing, housecleaning or whatever it is that you as a support person have to do to physically take care of the loved one. . . . This can be fairly difficult, but the solutions are also fairly obvious—you either do the extra work or arrange for someone else to do it.

"What is more difficult for the support person, however, and more insidious, is the inner turmoil that starts to accumulate on the emotional and psychological levels. This turmoil has two sides, one private and one public. On the private side, you start to realize that, no matter how many problems you personally might have, they all pale in comparison to the loved one who has cancer or some other life-threatening disease. So for weeks and months you simply stop talking about your problems. . . . You don't want to upset the loved one; you don't want to make it worse for them; and besides, in your own mind you keep saying, 'Well, at least I don't have cancer, my own problems can't be so bad.'"

Wilber goes on to explain in the article that the caregiver begins to realize that his or her problems, though minor in comparison to cancer, nonetheless persist and even worsen because now two problems exist: the original one plus the fact that you can't express and therefore solve the original problem.

"The problems magnify; you clamp the lid down harder; they push back with renewed strength. You start getting slightly weird. If you're introverted, you start getting little twitches; shortness of breath; anxieties start creeping up; you laugh too loud; you have an extra drink. . . . If you're introverted, there are times you want to die; if extroverted, times you want the loved one to die. . . . In any event, death hangs in the air; and anger, resentment, and bitterness inexorably creep up, along with terrible guilt about having any of those dark feelings."

Wilber's article then says that the only solution is to talk about those feelings. He mentions support groups and psychotherapy, but warns that the average person (including him) often waits to avail himself or herself of such services until "rather late in the game." Typically, most caregivers do what's most understandable, which is talk to friends, families, or associates. That's where the caregiver runs into the public problem.

"The public problem is this: as Vicky Wells (cofounder of Cancer Support Community of San Francisco) puts it, 'Nobody is interested in chronic.'" Wilber gives the following example: "I may come to you with a problem; I want to talk, I want some advice, I want some consolation. We talk; you are very helpful, kind and understanding. I feel better; you feel useful. But the next day, my loved one still has cancer; the situation is not fundamentally better at all. In fact, it might be worse. I don't feel good at all. Later, I happen to meet you again, and you ask how I'm doing. If I tell the truth, I say I feel awful. So we talk. You are again very helpful, kind and understanding, and I feel better . . . until the next day, when she still has cancer and nothing is really better.

"Sooner or later you find out that almost everybody not actually faced with this problem on a day-to-day basis starts to find it boring or annoying if you keep talking about it. All but your most committed friends start subtly avoiding you, because cancer *always* hangs over the horizon as a dark cloud, ready to rain on any parade. You may be perceived as a kind of chronic whiner, and people get tired of hearing the same old problem. Hence the observation, 'Nobody is interested in chronic.'"

Wilber meticulously and sometimes brutally outlines the danger of holding shameful thoughts and feelings inside. The caregiver not only imperils his or her own health, physical and/or mental, but also the health of the loved one. "It's not unusual for the support person to simply walk out of the situation. Treya and I have talked to women with cancer whose husbands lasted about six months, then walked, leaving them with the cancer, children, and no means of support."

Wilber further explains in "On Being a Support Person" how he coped, through support groups, psychotherapy, couples' counseling, and humor. It was almost too late.

"The most difficult emotional problems I had to deal with as a support person were resentment and self-pity. For about a full year I had a great deal of hatred and bitterness about the situation I was in. I had greatly curtailed or given up editorships at four different publishing concerns. . . . Worse yet, I had given up writing, which I considered my life-blood. You simply can't be a full-time support person and carry on a full-time career at the same time. I can't, anyway. . . . If I couldn't write, I saw no particular reason to carry on. Camus said the only really important philosophical question was whether or not to kill yourself. To be or not to be, that is the question. While contemplating this, I drank a lot of beer."

> *"When I went into the hospital, my daughter was there almost round the clock. But I worried that she wasn't exercising, and I wasn't strong enough to argue with her about it."*
>
> —E.C., lung cancer survivor

With much hard work and support, Wilber continued to care for his wife, realizing it was a choice he made of his own free will.

"I had made a fundamental choice to stay with this woman through thick and thin, no matter what, forever; to see her through this process come what may. But somewhere during the second year of the ordeal, I forgot about this choice, though it was a choice I was still making, obviously, or I would have left. . . . I had forgotten about my own choice, and therefore almost immediately fell into an attitude of blame and consequently self-pity. Somehow, this all became very clear to me."

Once he came to this realization, he experienced a change of heart and mind that did not necessarily make the choice any easier (or him any happier) but helped him cope day to day.

"So each day I re-affirm my choice. Every day I choose once again. This stops blame from piling up, and slows the accumulation of pity or guilt. It's a simple point, but actually applying even the simplest points in real life is usually difficult."

Wilber goes on to share coping strategies, which for him included making time to write, meditate, and engage in other activities involving self-care, which fed his soul while his caregiving contributes to his spiritual growth. He concludes:

"I still bitch and moan, I still get angry, I still blame circumstances, and Treya and I still half-kid (half-not) about holding hands, jumping off the bridge, and putting an end to this whole joke (fortunately, we're both cowards).

"And all in all, I'd rather be writing."

⊇⊇⊇

After Treya died, Wilber wrote in *Grace and Grit:*

"I had it all backwards: I thought my promise was how I would help her, whereas it was actually how she would reach and help me, again, and again, and forever again, as long as it took for me to awaken, as long as it took for me to acknowledge, as long as it took for me to realize the Spirit that she had come so clearly to announce. And by no means just me: Treya came for all her friends, for her family, and especially for those stricken with terrible illness. For all of this, Treya was present."

In the lap of love

When I was sick, my husband, David, cared for me perfectly, daily serving me warmth and compassion like a bowl of homemade chicken soup. He insisted on carrying the laundry up and down the stairs for months after my surgery; fielded well-meaning "How is Lori doing?" questions asked with furrowed brows that reminded him of all we had been through in the months before; cooked and cleaned, paid the bills, and cared for our teenaged son and four animals.

One of my biggest fears was that David would burn out. Because of the support of his employer, friends, and family, he was able to make it through. But my hope and my prayer is that, should I get sick again, he will avail himself of any and all resources to shore up his spirit and, more important, give a voice to his own pain.

Griffin taught me how to care for someone other than myself. As he lay dying of an untreatable brain tumor that must have caused unimaginable pain, I cradled him in my lap. Our veterinarian had come to our home to give him an injection so he could find final relief. David and I cried together. I was crying not just out of grief but out of gratitude. Griffin had taught me how to care for him and how to care for myself. It was a beautiful lesson I will never forget. My wish for you is that, as a caregiver, you learn that bittersweet truth for yourself.

20.

"I don't know if I'm cured, and bringing up my health can bring me down."

**Absence makes the heart grow fonder.
Out of sight, out of mind.**

—Two contradictory but reasonable idioms

WITH JUST ONE YEAR TO GO before graduation from UC Berkeley, Terry Healy, a handsome, healthy hunk who headed his fraternity, noticed what he thought was a pimple behind his right nostril. It took five weeks to determine that the lump was not a benign sign of stress known to many an undergrad, but a fibrosarcoma, a rare form of cancer that constitutes only one-half of 1 percent of all cancers. Relatively little is known about the disease, which can occur anywhere in the body, though not usually the face.

Terry's tumor was excised, and he needed neither chemo nor radiation, just a memory zap to forget those crazy two months. A small scar on his nose that made him look like he'd been in a fight was the only reminder, until six months later, when he felt a tingling in his cheek. Another mass had developed.

He was seen by a tumor board, a group of about fifteen oncologists and other medical specialists from diverse institutions who gather to review certain cases and collectively design the best course of action.

"I definitely felt like a lab specimen," Terry recalled. "There was no communication except gestures and body language. I saw shaking heads and things that really frightened me."

Terry's doctor came back into the examining room afterward and told him his "very serious situation" would require extensive surgery; his tumor may have reached his eye, and it would probably result in the loss of part of his nose and cheek, and perhaps other parts of his face.

During the next six years he underwent more than thirty operations, many to reconstruct his face, almost half of which had been removed.

He almost, but never quite, got used to the strange and sometimes cruel questions and remarks. "People would actually come up to me when I was riding BART [the Bay Area's rapid transit train system] and ask me what happened to my face."

"'Oh, I just KNOW that you're going to be cured!' That was the worst! I didn't know that at all. Of course I hoped for it. Disease and dying is a part of life for everyone. While I wanted people to be helpful, I wanted to deal with the situation as clearly and calmly as possible."

—D.P., cervical cancer survivor

One time he was sitting at a bar, and an older man bellied up and asked, "What in the hell happened to you?"

"I made a judgment that he was drunk and that he would not want to hear the truth," Terry laughed, "so I proceeded to tell him that I had been a DEA [Drug Enforcement Agency] agent who was working with border patrol agents in Texas, monitoring and surveying drug runners coming across the border. 'Out of nowhere there was gunshot,' I told him, 'and a bullet pierced through my cheek and nose!'"

Terry continued to tell the man that he had resigned from the agency to have his nose reconstructed. The man's response overwhelmed him.

"He thought I was a hero. He thought that I was everything that America stood for and said he admired me and I was courageous."

By that time, Terry had started to feel guilty about lying, but said he was too far along to stop. "The guy was eating it up. I'm sure he told all his buddies about me because he was fascinated by it, and we ended up talking for a long time."

Ultimately, that experience taught Terry that he needed to be honest with people. "That's the only way that people can learn from all these things. So today I make a conscious effort to tell children and adults exactly what happened to me so that they hear the truth from the outset."

Terry has told the entire truth in a book, *At Face Value: My Struggle with a Disfiguring Cancer*. He travels the United States as a motivational speaker, often appearing in news media. Although it's been almost twenty years since his diagnosis, a couple of things still bother him. One is being asked whether he's cured.

He was asked that during a radio station interview. "What are the odds of your being cured?" asked the host. "Is there a strong likelihood it won't come back?"

Terry said he never asked that question of his doctors, never wanted to know their answer. No two types of fibrosarcoma are alike, so the question didn't make sense to him.

"How are you supposed to respond to that?" Terry asked of the interviewer's questions. "To me that was never important and it shouldn't be. And doctors shouldn't offer that information up to patients. If I had been told when I was first diagnosed what I know now, I may have not behaved the same way. I was very impressionable."

Telling a patient they suffer from an incurable disease can be devastating. Asking them whether they are cured is something no one can ever know. If they believe they are cured, they will tell you that. If you love them, you will not question it.

Physician, heal thyself

Physician Ralph Berberich cured many children during his career as a pediatric hematologist (one who treats children with cancers of the blood such as leukemia). He found the work fulfilling, but after years of working with seriously ill children, he jumped at the chance to join a friend in establishing a new general pediatric practice. He was relieved after so many years of fighting cancer to fight the common cold and other relatively harmless ailments.

Dr. Berberich thought he was finished battling cancer. But twenty years later, it appeared in his own body. He wrote about it in his moving and powerful book, *Hit Below the Belt: Facing Up to Prostate Cancer*.

"The full impact of treatment goes well beyond facts. It is one thing to read about loss of hair. It's another to see your pubic hair thin to a point you haven't known since before you began adolescence, to see it almost gone. . . . It's one thing to read that you may lose sexual interest, and it is another to walk down the street, see a gorgeous woman, and have your mind register familiar sexual attraction but only in theory. . . . You are left feeling that your mind and desires are no longer connected to your body. How can books dealing with the facts of prostate cancer truly relate such sensations?"

"Here's the worst: 'So you're cured now?' What you want to say is, 'No, I have cancer for the rest of my life.'"

—E.K., lymphoma survivor

Dr. Berberich's book does so beautifully. And his words elegantly describe what it feels like to be asked whether you are cured of your cancer.

"People meet me today and ask whether I have completed treatment. I tell them that I have. They then often ask, 'So are you a survivor?' or 'Are you cured?' or 'Does this mean the cancer is gone?' No questions could be stranger when applied to cancer in general and to prostate cancer in particular. To both doctors and laymen, the word 'cure' means the illness is over for good. Cancer is never really over unless you die, have an autopsy, and are shown to be cancer free, in which case it is of no interest to you. The passage of time simply reduces the chance of recurrence, but it never completely eliminates it."

I can never know whether I'm cured

When someone asks me whether I'm cured, or whether I'm "okay," I usually answer, "As far as I know. As far as any of us know, we're cancer free until we find out otherwise."

I don't say that to disturb the person who has asked—to let him know that he, too, could have an undetected tumor growing stealthily within his own body—but to acknowledge that none of us can ever really know what the cells of our body may be doing.

Many patients act superstitiously because they feel out of control. Superstition is a way to abdicate control yet still feel in command, though that sounds contradictory. Saying, "I have been lucky" in no way guarantees I will continue to enjoy good luck, but if I knock on wood, so the gods may hear me, perhaps they will continue to help me live. If I say, "I am cured," I worry that the gods will show me who is boss and afflict me again. Primitive thinking, yes. Ridiculous thinking, yes. But the feeling? It's just as real as it is primitive and ridiculous.

"We look for signs, and it's natural because we have stopped living in the ordered, logical universe in which there is real causality in our daily lives," explained therapist Halina Irving. "One of the reasons we look for how to control the disease, is that we want the control, but another reason is that as human beings we come into the world with a need to find meaning, reason, cause, and effect in order to be able to live a predictable, rational life.

"When you are diagnosed with cancer," Irving continued, "you say, 'But I never ate fat and I never smoked and there's no family history of cancer and I'm such a good person, why did this happen to me?' That world has been turned upside down for us and that leaves room for superstition."

ट्टट्टट्ट

We also look to science and seek truth from the experts. I don't know a single patient who does not *love* for medical professionals to tell them they are cured. Doctor's words wield tremendous power.

I'll never forget the day when the head of pulmonology at the University of California at San Francisco, Dr. David Jablons, indicated I was cancer free.

"On the 'Are you cured now?' issue, every time they ask it, it drives home the point deep inside of you that you will never know."

—K.G., lung cancer survivor

"Lori, I believe you are cured of your cancer," he declared. Dr. Jablons was not my surgeon, but I had consulted him for a second opinion (I believe all cancer patients should receive at least a second and maybe a third opinion), and I had a great deal of respect for him. I had done enough research to know that the survival statistics for my kind of cancer, lung cancer, are not the best, but mine was caught early, and I am relatively young.

Also, some promising new treatments have recently become available.

Even so, I am a realist (full of hope, of course, but a realist nonetheless). Yet I absolutely loved it when Dr. Jablons said he believed I was cured.

That does not mean I *am,* of course, but it helps me look forward rather than back; it gives me more hope. When I have a down day, I try to replay Dr. Jablons's words in my mind; when I succeed, I eventually come back to believing that I may well live to see my son's children and maybe even mete out my retirement savings through my sixties, seventies, and eighties.

The cancer reminder diet

Patricia and Ewan were enjoying a dinner reunion with two of their oldest friends, Jackson and Paula, who had returned to the Bay Area for a visit after moving to Australia a year earlier. The conversation was animated, intelligent, and playful.

It had been almost two years since Patricia had undergone surgery, completing her treatment for lung cancer. "It was one of the first full days that I hadn't given even a thought to the disease that had darkened my soul like chimney soot," she recalled. "Even though the chimney will never be cleaned out completely, I had managed to escape it and was thoroughly relishing the light and air on the other side."

Then, just as she was about to dip her spoon into the chocolate pot de crème, it happened: the moment many cancer survivors fear as much as a child fears a shot in the rear.

"So, Patricia, when do you go to the doctor again?" Jackson asked. The question he had posed so gently blew a fuse in her head. She had finally managed to forget that she would have to return for medical tests every six months for the rest of her life, and suddenly, she found herself right back in the dark.

"You know, I'd rather not talk about that right now," Patricia told him matter-of-factly, instantly losing her appetite. She laughed now as she said, "On the positive side, at least he saved me from consuming those thousand-plus calories!"

Though she felt irritated, she knew Jackson did not—could not—understand the darkness that enveloped her. The evening of Viognier and port— plus a lack of experience with any traumatic suffering, as far as she knew—had rendered him emotionally clueless. But suddenly she felt stone cold sober. And she could not reclaim the levity and lightness of just one minute before.

Even though she had loved the fact that Jackson had inquired almost weekly about her health while she was undergoing treatment, she wanted to forget about the calamitous disease that had defined her as a victim for almost two years.

Think of September 11, 2001. Think of the 2004 tsunami that killed more than 150 thousand people and left millions more homeless. I have no idea what it feels like to be personally victimized by such overwhelming and unthinkable disasters, and I would never presume to know, but I do know what having cancer is like. For many of us, the internal implosion feels like an earthquake that cannot be seen and sometimes cannot be palpably felt, but that causes suffering resulting in deep depression and, according to a recent study, posttraumatic stress disorder in up to 19 percent of patients.

How you can help me live

I don't know if I am cured of my cancer, and I do not want you to ask me. I'd rather you not ask me specifically about my health at all. Instead, ask me how I am feeling today, and tell me I look younger than ever. If we are close enough, I will bring up the issue of being cured. I will bring up my fears—when and if I feel safe enough to do so.

Take me, take Terry, take Ralph Berberich, take Patricia, at face value. If we have a smile on our faces, you can assume we are feeling like we are cured, or that we have at least forgotten we had anything to be cured of. We might be feeling particularly hopeful—at least for the moment.

Love cures

Since we can never truly know what will help and what will hurt someone, how can we ever know what to say, ask, or do? I suppose the simple answer is, "We can't." But as H. L. Mencken said, "There is always an easy solution to every human problem—neat, plausible, and wrong."

The complex answer is that we can and we cannot know what our friend or loved one with cancer wants and needs. But we can always be sensitive.

"Our sensitivity consists of being able to hear what they want from us, what they need from us," said Halina Irving, "and to give that, and not to give what we believe they should want from us or need from us."

To discern what they want and need, we must call into play all of our senses and communication tools. We can pay attention to them, observing body language and facial expression.

We can talk to them and ask in a normal fashion, "How's it going?" Rather than asking, "How's your health?" or "How often do you have to go back to the doctor?" we can give people a choice of sharing any concerns, fears, or good news about their condition or not, talking instead about ordinary matters.

"When people ask if I'm cured, I feel like a liar if I say, 'Yes.' How do I really know? How does anyone know?"

—T.E., breast cancer survivor

We can ask how we might help; we can also ask forgiveness if we have caused any harm. We can say what most everyone in pain yearns to hear, whether they have cancer or any other disease or ailment and whether they are actively ill or recovering: *"I am here for you. I may not know exactly what to say or do, and if I mess up I apologize in advance, and I hope you forgive me. But I want you to know how much you mean to me."*

And, if it's true, we can add, "I love you." Then, if our friend or loved one grants permission, we can plant a kiss on their cheek and embrace them. Patting them very gently, we can whisper, "There, there . . . there, there . . . there, there."

That, quite simply, is what has helped me live.

afterword

IT'S 8:45 P.M. ON A SATURDAY NIGHT somewhere between Eugene and Chemult, Oregon, high in the Cascade Mountains. The railroad car floats along the tracks, and the comforting clack-clack-clack-clack grows louder and softer from minute to minute, depending on whether we are rounding a bend or heading straightaway.

Outside, a mountain, "Mount A-lotta-rock" according to our hilarious attendant, Donald, points like a pyramid, a symmetrical triangle with a background of clouds the color of Dreamsicles. Just to my left sits the most awe-inspiring beauty of all: my husband, David, studying the Amtrak schedule, hoping our train will arrive home late so we can enjoy as many minutes of this bliss as possible.

Suddenly, a tunnel. Darkness. Shock.

That's what it's like when someone asks me when my next CT scan is or whether I am cured of cancer.

Like going through an unfamiliar tunnel, you have no idea how long you will remain in the dark. And you have no idea what the world will look like when you come out the other end. You cannot know when darkness will overtake you again, shutting out all light. You may pop out for a hundred yards or so and delight in the beauty, only to enter another tunnel and hurtle through darkness again.

222

But on this day, David and I emerge from the tunnel, and the sun dips so low it turns almost red in the clean haze of the valley. Shining softly into my eyes, the burning star seems to say, "Don't worry. I will rise again tomorrow."

I look at my beloved husband, and then glance back at the orb that graces this planet with the miracle of its existence, day after day. I rest my head on David's shoulder and let my eyes close.

"Thank you," I smile, "for helping me live."

appendix

THE BIGGEST CHALLENGE IN WRITING this book was making it descriptive rather than prescriptive, or descriptive rather than judgmental. In other words, I wanted to describe what helped and hurt without making friends and loved ones feel guilty about things they may have said or done in the past, and without prescribing exact words or actions for the future. That's why I came up with "twenty things people with cancer want you to know," rather than "twenty things you should or shouldn't say or do."

That said, there are so many different circumstances, so many different kinds of cancer, and so many different stages that there was no way to cover everything. And I thought that many of you would be interested in specific situations, kinds of cancer, or issues.

Therefore, I have structured the appendix differently from the text of the book. This section includes special circumstances as well as lots of lists culled from friends, family, colleagues, and the survey I distributed (see next section), in addition to other interviews conducted and sources consulted during my process of research and writing. You will also hear from men and women who have written about their experiences expressly for this book or for magazines, journals, or other publications, and you will read excerpts from pamphlets and other materials.

This many-faceted guide is designed for easy reference. It is my hope that it helps you help your loved one live. May it also help improve your life and relationships!

I. The Survey

I wrote and distributed my survey with the goal of finding out what helped and what hurt real people who had survived cancer (as opposed to recording stories from medical and mental health professionals). I knew that each patient's experience would differ and that there would doubtless be hundreds of things people with cancer wanted others to know. I also knew the pool of respondents would be neither large nor controlled enough to deem the survey "scientific." I created it anyway, based on the twenty things I had heard most often and which resonated most strongly with me. Seventy-one people responded.

After an initial query as to the person's actual cancer diagnosis, the survey's next question was, "Has anyone ever said anything to you regarding your illness or condition that you think was meant to help you but in fact hurt you?" Most said "Yes." Two said they couldn't remember, and just seven said "No." And even those seven indicated later in the survey that they had been bothered or annoyed by something someone said to them. One man replied, "I really didn't want to hear about their other friends or family who had cancer. Not all of those people survived, and I didn't want to lump myself in with a group. . . . This was happening to ME, NOW."

Men more than women indicated they had not been hurt by other people's words. One caregiver whose wife had brain stem cancer, answered in the negative, but later he said, "My wife's doctor had some intern assistance. I distinctly remember one of them saying to my wife, 'Most people do not know how they are going to die. Now you do.' Those were the coldest and most upsetting words during this entire ordeal." The man went on to indicate that the worst thing was not the words that were spoken to his wife but the way most people avoided her.

Another respondent who said no one had said anything hurtful, later listed some remarks that had hurt her, including: "Oh, colon cancer. Don't worry, you'll be okay." She also wrote that "Good luck, I've gotta go now," bothered her because it made her feel that some people didn't have time for her.

A breast cancer survivor who answered no to the question, wrote, "One man saw the lines drawn on my neck for radiation when I had a low cut blouse on, and he had to walk away. Stupid man."

Still another who answered no wrote that she only told family and three friends because she was afraid of how people would react. Of her doctor, she wrote: "He was the most awful person I have ever encountered. I reported him to the head surgeon, who was wonderful and became my doctor. The awful doctor made my husband and myself feel terrible, ill, and like the world was falling apart. He was not nice, didn't show any sympathy at all."

Yet another said, "I couldn't deal with hearing about people who died from breast cancer or who had metastases. I did not join a support group because of my fear about hearing 'bad' news about how others were doing."

Another said, "No grim stories!" And another: "I hate to hear, 'You look tired.'"

One woman said she couldn't recall any hurtful remarks, but said she warned people about what to say. "My older sister had seen several friends through fatal cancer illnesses. And I told her I didn't want to hear anything about their struggles or demise."

A woman with melanoma wrote: "Most people are well-meaning, although uncomfortable in discussing diseases, and realizing this, nobody was able to hurt me (even though some people were real bunglers in their offers to help!)." She did, however, say she didn't want to hear survival statistics. And she ended with, "Friends show their true colors in time of need. Some can handle adversity; others cannot. Some are willing to help, no matter what is needed; others are not. At least now I know who my true friends are . . . and are not!"

One more who answered no to the question about whether anyone had done anything hurtful this way: "Actually, no, perhaps because I was so open with my cancer. I chose not to keep it a secret, but instead talked about it openly. Perhaps that made people feel more at ease with the subject and didn't create awkward moments where something hurtful might have been said. I still encountered people who didn't know how to respond but I tried to put them at ease. Their uncomfortable silence enabled me to talk to them and make them feel less uncomfortable considering the topic of cancer."

By the way, more than anything else, respondents said, first, they needed to forget and laugh; then, they wanted to be held in people's thoughts and prayers; then, they hoped to be helped without having to ask; and finally, they needed to simply know that people are there for them and that they will be listened to.

THE TEXT OF THE SURVEY

Help Me Live: 20 Things People with Cancer Want You to Know
Thank you for helping. I am a cancer survivor writing a book about what
to say and do to help people with cancer feel better. Although we all differ,
and what is a salve to one is a stab to another, most cancer patients and survivors agree that carefully chosen words and deeds can make a world of
difference. This survey is designed to find out what has helped and hurt
you; the purpose is to help others who come after us.

Since your responses will remain anonymous, please be as honest and
blunt as possible. If you'd like to be alerted when the book comes out,
please include your email address. Thank you again.
—Lori Hope

1. What kind of cancer do you or did you have, and when were you diagnosed? Feel free to provide as many details as you'd like.

2. Has anyone ever said anything to you regarding your illness or condition
   that you think was meant to help you but in fact hurt you?

3. If "yes," please explain. (Who, what, when, where, why, and most
   important, how it made you feel.)

4. Soon after you were diagnosed, what did you want or need or like to
   hear from people?

5. What did you NOT like or want to hear?

6. During treatment (please specify, e.g., surgery, chemo, radiation), what
   words did you like to hear, and which didn't you like to hear?

7. What about actions? If there were things friends or loved ones did that
   were helpful, please explain. Please explain things that were not helpful.

8. If there is one thing about you (thoughts, feelings) that you would like
   people who haven't had cancer to know, what would that be?

9. Here is the list of twenty-plus things many other cancer patients and survivors have said they want others to know. Please check the ones that
   apply to you. (*Note: These changed during the writing of this book.*)

☐ "Your words have more power over me than ever before."

☐ "How you listen to me can make a huge difference."

☐ "I am terrified."

☐ "I am more than my cancer."

☐ "I want you to help without my asking you to."

☐ "My moods change daily. Don't be afraid to ask [how I feel today]."

☐ "I need you to take care of yourself."

☐ "I need to know you accept my fears, even if they seem outrageous to you."

☐ "I need to know you realize you could be in the same boat as me."

☐ "I need to forget—and laugh!"

☐ "I need to know you are not judging me."

☐ "I want you to hold me in your thoughts and prayers."

☐ "I want you to understand if I don't call you back."

☐ "Once I've made my treatment decision, I don't want more advice."

☐ "Telling me to think positively can backfire."

☐ "I don't want to hear what's good about my cancer."

☐ "I will never know why I got cancer or if I'll get it again."

☐ "I need to know you're there."

☐ "Sometimes I am simply anxious and just want comfort."

☐ "I need to feel hope."

☐ "I need to feel useful."

Other (please specify).

If there's anything else you'd like to share, including your contact information, please do so here. Thank you again, and I wish you all the best!

    —Lori

II. Special circumstances

Not only are there more than two hundred different kinds of cancer, each with its own name and treatment, but every cancer has its own character and each cancer patient is different. Add time and space to the equation, and the possibilities for variation become infinite.

But, as humans, we like and need to categorize. The following section divides circumstances into those that distinguish a few cancer types and classes of treatments, age groups, and general stages of the disease. As in life, lines blur, white fades to gray before darkening to black, and forms overlap, but hopefully you will glean some insight or gain a new perspective.

SOON AFTER DIAGNOSIS

Most people with cancer experience shock, anger, and a sense of unreality such as they have never felt before. Terrifying and truly traumatic, cancer changes you in a way that is almost impossible to describe. As therapist Halina Irving, a cancer survivor herself, said, "It really feels like all at once, from one moment to the next, we've been plunged into the world of the absurd in which nothing makes sense, in which something has happened to us that goes against everything we ever believed would ever happen to us."

Irving said cancer patients are often told to think positively, but usually one's mind is too muddled to function in an even remotely normal fashion. "That person feels that there's a wild beast chasing them, and how can they think clearly and be proactive and feel positive when they have to escape from the clutches of death?"

The following, taken from *Taking Time: Support for People with Cancer and the People Who Care about Them,* by the National Cancer Institute, puts it well.

> "The first few weeks after the diagnosis are often the most emotional time of the entire cancer experience. Feelings change rapidly from day to day or even hour to hour. [Patients] may feel denial, anger, fear, stress and anxiety. [Their] sense of independence may seem threatened. At times [they] may also feel depressed, guilty or lonely."

Individuals who answered my survey said the following:

"Immediately after, I needed quiet time alone to listen to my heart and head (and have one good sob session). Then I just wanted my friends and family to be themselves; supportive but not fawning."

"At this point [two weeks after being diagnosed with Hodgkins], I don't feel like talking about the disease and while I want my friends and family to know I'll be okay, I'm running out of 'explaining' energy."

"The best thing I heard was from the first person I called. He started to say something, then stopped himself and said, 'What would be most helpful to you?' I started to apologize for being so upset, and he said, 'Don't apologize—you are going to feel all kinds of things at different times, and however you feel, it's ok.'"

"At first I needed time (at least twenty-four to forty-eight hours) to be alone with my thoughts and digest the reality of it all. I couldn't talk to many people because I was constantly crying, so I had my husband call family, and then one girlfriend would let all the rest know. Eventually the word got out, and I was able to focus on gathering information and making decisions."

"Suddenly, you're a mere mortal, and the possibility of death is real. There is also a sense of betrayal . . . how could my body give out on me this way?"

DURING TREATMENT

When I was a medical reporter, I remember once using the term "side effects" when interviewing a doctor about a pharmaceutical treatment. He corrected me, saying something like, "There are not *side* effects, there are *effects*, plain and simple." In other words, a treatment's side effect can be an entrée in itself. A side effect may exert more power than an actual treatment.

I was fortunate that my only cancer treatment was surgery, and I suffered few "side" effects. But many others endure treatments such as chemotherapy and radiation in addition to or in place of surgery, and they suffer not only physical but psychological effects that exacerbate the pain or difficulty of treatment.

Surgery

When I was younger, the idea of someone cutting into my body did not frighten me much. But many of us, as we age, become more leery of letting someone cut into our flesh. I was, to put it bluntly, absolutely terrified. Books and tapes about preparing for surgery through meditation and visualization helped calm me, and I would recommend buying such resources (see resources section) for anyone who expresses fear about going under the knife (after asking permission to do so, of course).

Here are some quotes from responses to my survey about what helped and hurt people about to undergo surgery for cancer.

> "During my time of surgery, I wanted to hear about quick and easy recoveries. I wanted to hear how unlikely it was that I would develop lymphadema [painful swelling of the upper arm]. I wanted to hear great stories about my surgeon. Post-op I wanted to hear what great progress I was making and how quickly I was recovering. I wanted to hear that the pain I was experiencing was normal."

> "I liked hearing that it was normal to be so very tired after the surgery because I could do very little without being exhausted."

> "I don't even believe in God, per se, but I love being prayed for."

> "My wonderful surgeon kept apologizing for the big scar I would have. I told him I didn't care because I wanted to be clear and healthy . . . and wake up with my leg still attached to my body. He was impeccable—the scar is big but it is perfect."

> "During treatment (surgery in my case), I wanted to hear how well I was doing, how good I looked, how strong I was. I did not want to hear how skinny I had gotten, or how scared they were for me. That just made it worse."

> "After surgery, it was good to hear 'You're doing great!'"

Hospitalization

A friend of mine who was diagnosed with cancer almost refused surgery because he had heard so many horror stories about hospitals, but what I encountered more than stories about infections or poor nursing care were tales of people receiving unwanted visitors who overstayed their welcome or talked incessantly or too loudly.

Most people who are hospitalized for cancer surgery or treatment appreciate being asked whether they want visitors. It can be difficult for them to ask visitors to leave once they have arrived, so it's important to ask how long the patient would like you to stay.

Whether you visit or not, almost all patients appreciate flowers, plants, and greeting cards. But be careful about bringing books. Again, it's good to ask. One friend of mine who was hospitalized for several weeks while undergoing treatment for leukemia said she received many more books than she had the time or energy to read, and it made her feel bad that she could not tell the gift-bearers she had read what they had so generously given her.

If you do visit, try to remain as calm as possible. People who are sick become more sensitive to movement, as illustrated in this story told to me by Susan Chernak McElroy, *New York Times* best-selling author and speaker/comedienne extraordinaire.

"There are silences that are healing and there are silences that are toxic, and I've had them both. When I had my second extreme makeover [Susan had head and neck cancer and surgery that made her neck swanlike albeit scarred], I told nurses I didn't want anyone to come in and visit me, because no one who came in to see me came into that place with a healthy silence.

"This is about how it's going for me: You're laying there plugged in, wishing they gave you Metamucil, and a guest comes in."

Susan took a deep breath before spewing out the following: "'Hey, Susan!Lookin' great!How you feelin'?I see the TV's on.Want the TV on or want me to turn it off?Want a magazine,book?No?Fine.No magazine.No book.Want the window open?No it doesn't open?They afraid you'll jump out?So how have you been? Oh, you're crying! I'll come back another time!'

"That's why I didn't have guests come in. It's kind of like having your bone marrow sucked out and put in a bowl.

"When you're laying there healing, you're supposed to cheer them up; you're supposed to say, 'I'm just fine! I'll make you feel fine, and you'll make me feel fine, and we'll all just feel just fine!'"

One woman who answered my survey who had been hospitalized said she liked visitors to do the following: "Sit, let me sleep in their presence, read to me, tell me the banalities of their life instead of asking me to rehash my violent hospital experience over and over."

Chemotherapy

Many cancer patients fear chemotherapy more than any other treatment. Although it can prevent suffering and save lives, it also can devastate the intestinal tract and stomach by killing normal fast-growing cells as well as cancer cells.

I cannot describe what it's like to undergo chemo myself, but I have been told it is like the worst imaginable flu. Think of a time you have been horribly nauseated. Add to that losing your hair and you can imagine how much you would need extra TLC!

Here's an excerpt of an email my friend Laura's husband, Dan, sent out while she was undergoing chemo and lost her hair. Laura cherished the note!

"She is still as pretty as ever. Some people would kill for such a lovely shaped head. She now has a choice of three wigs. She is blonde one day. A brunette the next and a redhead the next day. When we are out I don't recognize her. Who knew cancer could be this sexy? I would have bought her wigs long ago!"

What follows are suggestions from people who answered my survey regarding chemotherapy.

"What I wanted to hear during chemo was, 'We will get you through this,' or, 'We're almost done'!"

"During chemo, a good friend and neighbor brought some homegrown tomatoes. At a time when I could not eat very much, these tasted so good!"

"I appreciated jokes about the chemo (such as calling the bright blue stuff the '7-11 slurpy blue chemo') and any comments about the chemo as helping to fight the cancerous cells. Referring to the chemo as toxic in general was not helpful. I did not need to think of it as beating me up. It was beating up the cancer more, and that's what I needed to focus on."

"During chemo, it hurt to hear, 'It's only hair.'"

"What I didn't want to hear: 'That wig looks *really* nice. It doesn't look a bit like you, but it looks really good!'"

"A classmate in the master's program I was in kept insisting that he was going to pull my wig off so he could see how my head looked. I wanted to slap him."

"Well, I got VERY tired of people telling me what a beautifully shaped skull I had. Sometimes the little things get to you the most. But someone could tell me I looked just dreadful and I could accept that—it was true."

"I had a long talk with a friend who is a homeopathic practitioner. He kept telling me that the chemo was poison and encouraging me to deny it and try some nontoxic treatments. It didn't help me at all. My choice wasn't respected, and I was left with a sinking suspicion that I may be choosing to poison myself."

"I didn't like it when people were constantly asking me if I had lost my hair. And 'Are you throwing up?' and wanting full details of my nausea."

"Several well-meaning friends told me horror stories about huge weight gains . . . and having to self-inject with meds (in the stomach) and terrible nausea. None of those things happened to me or anyone I met while going through chemo and radiation. EVERYONE is different and reacts differently to the medications."

"I didn't like the comments that trivialized or denied how awful I felt some days right after chemotherapy. I'd hear comments like, 'But you look soooo good.' They were meant to be polite, but they just irritated me because comments like that suggested that I was somehow lying about how bad I felt, insinuated that if I looked good, I must have felt good, too."

Radiation

Conventional cancer treatments—surgery, chemotherapy, and radiation—have been referred to as "slash, poison, and burn." But radiation does not always cause a burning sensation; sometimes it just saps energy, and other times people experience no negative side effects at all. Those who answered my survey indicated they appreciated sensitivity, honesty, and openness when they were undergoing radiation.

> "The doctors downplayed the side effects of radiation, minimizing them even as I was suffering them. 'That will go away' was not helpful. More helpful would have been advice about coping."

> "Once I decided to go ahead with radiation, I didn't want to hear stories about how dangerous radiation is or how it causes cancer. I wanted coaching on how to see radiation as a positive thing (think of the radiation as sunlight, shining on your breast and healing it)."

> "Unhelpful words: 'Oh, radiation treatment is really no big deal; you'll feel a little tired and have a mild sunburn. Take a little Ibuprofen if you feel pain.' I experienced third-degree burns with sloughing and open, weeping wounds that would not heal; I needed to take narcotics. I was 'fatigued' for a year and a half after radiation. Every woman's experience is unique, and don't dismiss the serious risk and potentially bad outcomes because it happens only one in a hundred. When you're that one, you are angry that you weren't properly informed."

> "Unhelpful: 'But you look so healthy'—like just because you have your hair and don't look sickly, the radiation is nothing."

WORKPLACE ISSUES

When I was diagnosed with cancer, I was self-employed, so I did not have to worry about losing my job. I did, however, fear losing my income. I was fortunate to feel fully supported by my principal client, Give Something Back Business Products. The owners and the human resources director made it clear to me that there would be work waiting for me after my recovery, and I cannot express enough how much that helped me. It did not take me long to spend a large part of my savings during the five months of my illness, treatment, and recovery, and I needed to know I would be able to earn a living again. I also needed to know that my boundaries would be respected: I knew I would not be able to work with as much vigor as I had before, at least initially. Again, I was fortunate to be supported so firmly by Give Something Back.

As indicated in the following survey responses, not everyone is as lucky.

"I was diagnosed with calcifications in my right breast, which turned out to be precancerous. The growth was a high grade, so I had to have a mastectomy. I had a coworker who was supportive at the beginning, but once I came back to work and had ongoing treatments, she completely forgot what I had gone through and felt I should put my job first instead of my appointments. I think that's just the way her personality is, but it bothered me, so I told her my life came first. Also, when I was off work for my leave of absence, she reminded me how I should hurry back to work or my position wouldn't be available. I told her my health came first, and I could take up to a year if I needed it. I stood up for myself, but I didn't need her to stress me out about my job."

"When I returned to work, my girlfriends there were so protective. They wanted to make sure I wasn't working too hard and that people didn't come up and say dumb things. They were my gatekeepers, so to speak, and they did an effective job."

"I went back to work afterward, and most people seemed to ignore what I was going through. I think they were uncomfortable asking, but acknowledging that I was going through some tough times would have been nice."

"The day I returned to the office after my second chemo treatment and wearing my wig for the first time, my boss asked me, 'How many more days do you think you will need to take off? We want to support you, but we have a business to run.' At that moment I decided that I needed the company for my paycheck and my insurance. I decided that I would look for a new job once I was past my treatment."

"My supervisor asked me how long it was going to be until I was back to the level that they had come to expect from me. This was about a month after my eight-month treatment course.

Keep in mind that prior to learning about my cancer, I was doing the work of two people, running two separate programs. I was working to give myself a sense of normalcy, and she was concerned with my productivity and her bottom line. I felt betrayed by someone who continually had told me that she would do anything for me. I guess that was true when it was convenient."

"I needed people to let me handle my emotional reaction to the diagnosis the way I wanted to react. At first, for example, I tried to explain to my employer that she needed to get someone in so I could train them to take over my duties. I told her we all needed to hope for the best, but still plan for the worst. . . . She didn't want to hear that. She didn't want to hear that I might not survive . . . but at the time I needed her to."

DEPRESSION

Cancer treatment may change the way an individual's brain works, actually *causing* depression. According to the National Institute of Mental Health (NIMH), studies indicate that about 25 percent of people with cancer experience depression, yet only 2 percent of cancer patients in one study were receiving antidepressant medication. "Despite the enormous advances in brain research in the past 20 years," reports an NIMH fact sheet on depression and cancer, "depression often goes undiagnosed and untreated."

The paper continues, "Persons with cancer, their families and friends, and even their physicians and oncologists may misinterpret depression's warning signs, mistaking them for inevitable accompaniments to cancer. Symptoms of depression may overlap with those of cancer and other physical illnesses."

The NIMH says treatment for depression can not only help people feel better and cope more effectively with the cancer treatment process, it can also help enhance survival. "Support groups, as well as medication and/or psychotherapy for depression, can contribute to this effect." *(Note: For people who shy away from support groups or who are too ill to attend, there are numerous online and telephone support groups that have helped many cancer patients. See the resources section.)*

As Lawrence LeShan, PhD, told me, there are two types of depression, and they overlap. "There's realistic depression and neurotic depression. Most cancer depression is realistic. Most people who get cancer were raised when getting cancer was an absolute disaster.

"With neurotic and psychological depression, the best thing is antidepressives. With realistic depression you may occasionally use antidepressants as a startup point, a jump-start. You say, 'All right, lets get some action' lets do this.'"

LeShan considers antidepressants useful to jump-start treatment, but says medications cannot change depressive illness. "They make the immune system function better because you feel better, because they mask the depression. That masking is marvelous, because then you start acting in such a way that you find more enthusiasm in your life."

If a cancer patient resists taking medications, LeShan suggests saying something like the following to your friend or loved one: "You seem depressed; you don't feel like moving. It's not good for you. You may not feel like you care that much right now, but if there's something you would like to do if you weren't depressed, I'll go with you the first time. If it's too much trouble to get your car out of the garage, I'll take it out for you the first time, then I'll get the hell out of your way."

Again, what is most important is to be there for your loved one. He or she probably does not want to be told what to do, but gentle suggestions made with love (after asking permission to make such suggestions, of course) may be deeply appreciated.

For more about depression, see "Soon after Treatment Ends," page 223.

BREAST CANCER

I had two first cousins who had breast cancer in their thirties and forties. As you read in the preface, I thought I understood cancer. But you cannot ever understand what it's like to have your body turn against itself until it does. And when it threatens a part of you that is private yet public, precious yet not necessary for life itself, sexual yet not necessary for sexual relations, it gets very complicated indeed. Again, all women experience breast cancer differently, but I think it is safe to say that most believe the subject should be treated with extra care. Special care should be taken when asking questions and offering suggestions such as the following ones given by my survey respondents.

"'Did your mother have breast cancer?' When I responded, 'Yes,' the people (this happened at least five times) visibly sighed in relief that there was a reason I had this."

"[It was unhelpful when] someone suggested I not have reconstructive surgery following my mastectomy so I could make a political statement by having no breast. Also unhelpful was: 'There are so many things they can do for breast cancer now.' While it may be true that there are more treatments than before, breast cancer still kills over forty thousand women in this country per year, plus thousands and millions more all over the world."

"I wanted my husband to say he would love me just as much without a breast and I was still beautiful to him. I did not want people to say things that made me feel sorry for myself."

"I talked to one person who said, 'Why don't you just have a mastectomy?' like your breasts don't mean anything. I know doctors aren't there to handle your feelings, but every time I'd express concern about losing my breasts or saving my breasts I'd hear, 'Well you really should consider a mastectomy,' but I was never told why. Why does it flow off the tongue so easily like it's an easy thing to do?"

PROSTATE CANCER

As with any form of cancer, it is important to ask permission before asking personal questions, but in the case of prostate cancer, it is particularly important since it can impact a man's sexuality.

As prostate cancer is a male disease, this section relates to "Gender Issues," page 218. And for more information, please refer to Dr. Ralph Berberich's excellent memoir about his own bout with prostate cancer (see resources section). The following statements made by survey respondents who survived the disease provide some interesting insight, as well.

"After the surgery to remove the prostate, I wanted to hear, 'You are cancer free.' I got that response from my doctor after I had a follow-up blood test to check my PSA levels. Every indication was that the cancer had been completely removed."

"I didn't like hearing that my postoperative recovery could be as long as six months to a year. Dealing with incontinence and erectile dysfunction was tough."

"I didn't want to hear the horror stories of someone who had died from prostate cancer. Some people like to revel in the gruesome details. I chose to avoid those kind of people."

LUNG CANCER

Few people who have had lung cancer want to be asked whether they smoke or used to smoke; no one needs to be told they should quit. Hold your tongue. Don't add insult to injury. Everyone knows smoking is dangerous; bringing up that reality can be injurious as well. In fact, a recent study by the University of Oxford in the United Kingdom showed that the stigma attached to patients with lung cancer can have a serious negative impact on their physical and mental health.

The study found the stigma, shame, and blame caused some patients to conceal their illness, which sometimes resulted in their not seeking all the required treatment for their disease. Many of the patients, especially those who had never smoked or who quit years before their diagnosis, felt unjustly blamed for their illness. Said one, "People automatically think you've brought it on yourself."

If someone with lung cancer has never been a smoker, you will likely learn that without having to ask.

RARE CANCERS

It's important to do research on cancer in general and on a friend's rare type of cancer, in particular, before asking about it. It will help you avoid asking questions that could hurt, such as, "Aren't there some clinical trials you could enroll in?" Most rare cancers receive few research dollars. Asking about clinical trials can be a hope killer.

As one woman with leiomyosarcoma—a quickly mutating form of cancer that responds to one chemotherapeutic agent for a short while, but then stops—told me, "Friends think since you're having chemo you'll be fine, but no, it only works for a few months. Sometimes you just want to say to them, 'How in the hell do you know?' Basically you know people are trying to be nice, but it can be very hurtful."

CHILDREN AND CANCER

Talking with children who have cancer is like talking with anyone else, but it is of vital importance that you ask the child's parent for permission first. Once a mom, dad, or guardian grants permission, therapist Halina Irving recommends saying something like the following to the child:

"You don't have to, but I want you to know that if you have concerns, anxieties, pain, or worry that you need to talk about that I'm here—able and willing and loving to listen. You don't have to talk to me, but it's okay. Most people find it helpful to talk, but it doesn't have to be now; it can be whenever you like, if you like."

For more information, see *Armfuls of Time: The Psychological Experience of the Child with a Life-Threatening Illness* by Barbara M. Sourkes, PhD (see resources section).

GENDER ISSUES

Again, I turned to Halina Irving for insight into whether to approach males and females differently. She told me she and a male therapist once co-facilitated a support group for women with cancer and their significant others. At first, he worked with the men and she worked with the women; then they brought them together. This is what she observed (being careful to stress that she was making a generalization):

"Men, I think, are more threatened by feelings that make them feel vulnerable because they equate them more with weakness than women do. They are more prone to want to forget about [cancer], both if it happens to them and if it happens to their wives or significant others. They think, 'It's over; it's in the past, get over it, forget it.'" Irving said men demand that of themselves as well as of the people in their lives; they see continued emotional bouts as signs of dwelling or wallowing and of negative thinking. She said it was more difficult to work with men.

"The only way we were able to get men to come to our group was by telling them they were coming to help their wives, not that it would help them. In that way, I think you need to work hard to keep that in mind when you deal with a man, because a man needs to feel that he can be able to save face more than a woman. A woman has that tendency too, but not as much, and will not experience having the emotions of having to be shamed or to lose face the way men experience it."

"So men want to be kept in denial more?" I asked.

"They have a greater need not to allow themselves to feel the normal feelings that go with a diagnosis of cancer, because it makes them feel weak or vulnerable. After all, men more than women believe they're supposed to solve everything, and they're supposed to be goal-oriented; they're supposed to solve things through action, and so it's very hard for them when there is no action possible. For them passivity is harder than for women."

In my experience, men don't like to be coddled as much as women like to be comforted. Dr. Lawrence LeShan said to me, "For God's sake, don't wrap me in cotton batting and say, 'You poor dear thing, let me take care of you!' More people have died suffocated in cotton batting than from cancer," LeShan joked.

YOUNG ADULTS

Most of us think of cancer as an older person's disease. But according to recent findings by the Division of Preventive Oncology at Cancer Care in Ontario, Canada, more young adults (in their twenties and thirties) are being diagnosed, especially with brain, testicular, and thyroid cancer and non-Hodgkin's lymphoma.

For more information about helping young adults with cancer, contact Vital Options International (www.vitaloptions.org and see resources section), a nonprofit cancer communications, support, and advocacy organization whose mission is to facilitate a global cancer dialogue.

The following words written by cancer survivor Kairol Rosenthal, author of *Mortality Bites,* presents a very clear picture of what it's like to have cancer as a young adult:

> I was diagnosed with cancer four years ago at age twenty-seven. Receiving a diagnosis in your twenties and thirties is no better or worse than being diagnosed during later decades; it is simply a hell of a lot different. When I was diagnosed I had no boyfriend, no husband, no children. No relatives living nearby. I lived alone in a disheveled three-story walk-up, paying cheap rent and writing on my fire escape until three o'clock in the morning. I was sending off manuscripts, applying to graduate school, rehearsing, performing, and barely surviving off my part-time administrative job. I was developing deep friendships and establishing myself in San Francisco, a city I had moved to

just one year before. I was dating, and, well, sleeping around.

While in my prediagnosis life I was a woman hammering out my artistic goals, I was also the poster child of instability. This instability is the trademark of life as a young adult. Though unpredictability and newness manifest differently in each of us, most are grasping to define themselves financially, romantically, geographically, or professionally. Add cancer to the equation and you have a situation that looks exponentially different from your parents' and grandparents' cancer. You have the same disease but an inherently different lifestyle than the older men and women perched next to you on the couch at your average cancer support group. You are the age of their children and grandchildren. You begin to suspect that out of all the people in the group living with cancer, yours is the only nightstand that is cluttered with orange prescription bottles, condoms, and a boxed set of *Sex and the City*.

Most people I know in their twenties and thirties are not on a first-name basis with their pharmacist, nor do they scan their disability insurance policy with a fine eye, and none have their primary care physician's number programmed into speed dial. In the midst of my cancer, I found myself surrounded by peers who had the luxury of not facing illness and death each morning when they looked in the mirror.

I want people who do not have cancer to know that contemplating mortality is not a lesson reserved for our elders or for those of us who live with life-threatening diseases. Becoming intimately acquainted with your own mortality is your responsibility as an alive and aware person and also your duty as a friend to anyone who is facing death on a daily basis.

Some have placed my proximity to death on a pedestal, as though I am a beacon who, at a young age, is bestowed the honor of looking the scary beast of death straight in the face. I want people who live free of cancer to know that everyone has the choice to become deeply familiar with their own mortality. Most young adults can't imagine death as clearly or as vividly when they are healthy, riding the subway home from work or going to yoga, as they can if they are laying in bed hooked up to a morphine drip. It is your responsibility nonetheless.

It is your duty to look death squarely in the face, not as a gesture of sympathy, and not only because it is reality, but because it is too large a task for people living with cancer to carry on our own. Young adults living with cancer are not, and never chose to be, the death and dying ambassadors from our generation. I have had peers explain to me that I have to think about death because I have cancer and may be dying, but they don't have to think about death because they are young and death is not yet knocking on their door. My response: We are all dying. Once you face this sharp and weighty reality, you will be able to sit beside your young friends who have cancer with less fear, less discomfort, less nervousness. You will erase the boundary that divides us and them, the sick and the well, the fortunate and the less fortunate. From this place, you can provide the very simple comfort of compassion that people living with cancer desperately want.

WOMEN IN THEIR CHILDBEARING YEARS

Chemotherapy can wreak havoc with a woman's reproductive system, and it is important to understand the challenges faced by premenopausal women so you can be as supportive as possible. The following was written by a friend of mine who asked that I not share her name.

> When I got the final results of my biopsy for non-Hodgkin's lymphoma, it confirmed I had a more aggressive form than originally indicated, so I was put into chemotherapy a few days later. There were no discussions about harvesting my eggs or doing anything else to preserve my fertility. I was told later there simply wasn't time. At thirty-seven, I was unmarried but still hoping to have children. At the very least, I did not want that possibility taken away from me. My doctors, while kind, were understandably less concerned about my fertility than about getting rid of my cancer. It was difficult for me to hear about the fertility problems of friends because that was the biggest problem in their life. For me, it was simply a side effect of my treatment. I became one of those people who have a problem so big that something like having children would be considered a luxury. I was supposed to be content just to be alive.
>
> My periods stopped sometime around the second course of chemo. I went through the process pretty smoothly, rarely

showing any signs of sadness or fear. In the middle of chemo, I went to Stanford University for a second opinion. The doctor commented on how well I was responding, but she suggested extending the number of rounds because of the large size of my original tumor. I knew that with each successive round, my chances of getting my menstrual cycle back would diminish. But I knew I could not consider that in my decision. She told me that at my age, the chances of remaining in permanent menopause were fifty-fifty. And even if I did get my cycle back, the damage to my eggs and follicles could leave me sterile. After the appointment, I went out to lunch with my parents and burst into tears over a plate of pasta. My hormone levels put me squarely in menopause. I would joke about my hot flashes with women in their fifties.

I saw my gynecologist and a reproductive endocrinologist to discuss hormone replacement therapy. But about a month or so later, I started feeling a familiar sensation I usually got at the onset of my period. The day it began, I had not been so excited since I was fourteen and a half and was convinced I was the last girl in high school to menstruate. After getting monthly periods for about nine months, I returned to my gynecologist for some additional tests. I found out that not only had my hormone levels returned to normal but that there was every indication that I was ovulating. Once again, I burst out in tears. I do not know if I will have children, or at least bear them, considering I am near the end of my biological clock. I am even considering the possibility of having them on my own [as a single parent]. But my point is that I feel blessed that I still may have a choice—that cancer has not taken this away from me. While nobody said this with anything other than good intentions, I get the sense from other people that they feel I should not worry about this and just be grateful to be alive. I am grateful. But I think the reason that I get so upset is that it hits me on a deep level, as a cancer survivor and as a woman. I let my emotions go about my fertility and hormonal problems in a way I can't about the cancer.

PARENTS WITH CANCER

When I was diagnosed with cancer, The Cancer League, a volunteer organization of women impacted by cancer, donated a grant in my honor to the East Bay Agency for Children and the Women's Cancer Resource Center to support a program to help teens whose parents have had cancer. I was deeply touched, heartened, and grateful, not only because my son would be able to attend the group but because other youth would benefit from the support. I knew that although the tendency among friends and loved ones of people with cancer is to offer support to the person who actually has the disease, most cancer patients who have children know their sons and daughters need just as much help. You can help your loved one by searching out programs that support children and teens online as well as face-to-face, and the following comments from my survey respondents point out practical ways to offer support.

> "I wanted parents of my kids' friends to perhaps offer to do the driving to sports and offer to pick up the practice schedules at parent meetings and that sort of thing."

> "Food was helpful for my family . . . but not always casseroles, which most children don't eat. My kids could have used more distractions. People should have been inviting them to the movies and fun activities just to get them out of the house."

> "Helpful were the friends and family who provided babysitting for my two-year-old, food, and housecleaning and support for my husband."

> "I appreciated people who offered to help get my kids, who were quite young then, from place to place."

SOON AFTER TREATMENT ENDS

I felt wholly loved and cared for during my cancer treatment and exhilarated to be alive right afterward. But soon I began a slow slide into a well of depression that went unnoticed until I opened my eyes and could see nothing but black in my present and future. Instead of experiencing terror, as I had upon my diagnosis, I felt numb, dead inside. How could I feel that way after being given the gift of survival?

Depression is common among cancer survivors, as are concerns about recurrence. *Facing Forward, Life after Cancer Treatment: A Guide for People Who Were Treated for Cancer,* by the National Cancer Institute, states that "Worrying about the cancer coming back (recurring) is normal, especially during the first year after treatment. This is one of the most common fears people have after cancer treatment."

Sometimes cancer survivors are surprised by reminders, says the guide. "For example, one person said he used to go to a particular restaurant during chemo because the milkshake it served was the only thing he could stand to eat. After treatment, he found he had to stop going to the restaurant because it reminded him of treatment and made him 'sick to his stomach.'"

It's important to be sensitive to such reminders and to other issues, as indicated by the following comments from my survey.

> "Mostly, after time goes by, after treatments are over, one wishes to find normal life again, and sometimes people don't let you forget, by always acting as if you are fragile."

> "No matter how one handles the decision making or treatment, this is a journey—even after the treatment is over, there are continuing checkups, physicals, etcetera that bring back the dark times and fears. Lots of things can trigger thoughts of metastasis or recurrence—a poor bone density test, a new pain, a change in cholesterol levels even."

> "I wanted people to ask how I was doing, but not to indicate they were asking about my cancer. Sometimes I was able to forget I had had cancer and didn't want to be reminded by their acting overly concerned."

LONG-TERM SURVIVORS

During the first year following my treatment, I did not think I would ever feel "normal" again. Indeed, days can now pass without my thinking about the disease at all. But the experience, the memories, and the fears remain and can arise quickly, no matter how many months or years have passed. As the booklet, *Facing Forward, Life after Cancer Treatment: A Guide for People Who Were Treated for Cancer,* by the National Cancer Institute, indicates, "Even years after treatment, some events can cause you to become worried about your health. These may include: follow-up visits; anniversary events (like the day you were diagnosed or had surgery or ended treatment); illness of a family member; symptoms similar to the ones you had when you found you had cancer; the death of someone who had cancer."

The following comments from my survey provide additional insights.

"Many people, friends, and family have indicated that 'it's over now' since I'm four years post-diagnosis. Well, it's not over, as I still have fear of recurrence, which is near impossible to discuss with anyone outside the 'cancer circle.'"

"I still fear cancer, and it's still got a grip on my emotions. It is hard to share your fears, especially when 'healthy' people can't understand the longevity of them."

"There was a time when I thought I would think about my cancer every day and now, thirteen years later, I don't. But it still intrudes at times, and then I'm right back there. So recognize the pain and try to give some quiet hope, but, of course, be careful how you say this."

FOR THOSE OF FAITH

My belief in God, or the power of love that I consider my god, strengthened during my bout with cancer. Although faith is not something you can impart to anyone, and many feel betrayed by God when they or someone they love receives a cancer diagnosis, spirituality of any kind—which can include a walk in the forest, meditation, or other forms of self-care—may be helpful, as indicated by the following comments from cancer survivors.

"When I first left the doctor's office, upon being referred to a surgeon to evaluate the lump in my breast, my level of anxiety rose considerably. I got in the car, and I began to pray, intending to ask God for a benign lump. Immediately, even before I could utter this prayer, I felt an almost physical support and assurance that, no matter what, God would carry me through whatever was to be. I was literally unable to pray this prayer, and instead it became a prayer of thanksgiving that our God was in complete control, whatever the outcome. That proved to be the case. I prayed through every radiation treatment, asking God to be with the technicians, to direct the rays to the exact spot where they should go, and to avoid places where they should not. I had no problem with the treatment."

"I am a Christian, and my faith sustained me through the entire process. I found great comfort that I was not alone even when I was physically alone with my inner thoughts. I also believe that many prayers were said for me, and there is power in prayer."

"I wanted reassurance that I would move past this and live a long, happy, healthy life. I wanted to be reassured that despite this bad bump in the road, God would walk me through this. I wanted unconditional love and understanding about what I was going through."

"A friend called with some scripture, which I held onto like a lifeline, Jeremiah, NIV Version: 'For I know the plans I have for you, says the Lord; plans to prosper you and not to harm you; plans to give you a future and a hope.' I also had an abundance of Christian friends praying for me. They sent me cards and notes, which I kept up on the kitchen counters and overflowed into the dining room area. I kept these up all through radiation treatments, as a visual reminder that all these people were upholding me in prayer."

END-OF-LIFE ISSUES

Talking with and supporting people in the process of letting go of life can be one of the most difficult challenges of all. An article about dying by Elizabeth Ford Pitorack, director of the Hospice Institute of Western Reserve in Cleveland, was quoted in the *New York Times*. In "Facing Up to the Inevitable, In Search of a Good Death," columnist and author Jane Brody wrote honestly and eloquently about Pitorack's findings.

"As someone nears the end of life, it is not unusual to turn inward and become less communicative, even as much as three months before death. Ms. Pitorak noted that loved ones should not confuse this withdrawal with rejection. Rather, she said, it reflects the dying person's need to leave the outer world behind and focus on inner contemplation.

"Patients who ask whether they are dying should be answered honestly and reassured that those left behind will be well, which Ms. Pitorak says is more helpful than telling patients, 'You can go now.'" [You can access the entire article online by going to www.nytimes.com or www.deathwithdignity.org.]

Therapist Halina Irving offered some important insights, as well: "Even people who are dying, you can see they find comfort when they feel understood and when their feelings are being accepted. That relates back to that whole issue of the connection with another person, which is the only thing that gives us solace and comfort.

"I have talked with dying people who have felt so alone because every time they've tried to talk about the fact that they are dying and they want to take care of business—they want to say their final good-byes—their families feel threatened and then say, 'Don't say that, don't talk about it, don't talk negatively,' and they then die isolated and alone."

The following, excerpted from *The Caregivers Handbook,* by Jim and Joan Boulden, provides more crucial information:

> Dying people are often honest and open to an extent rarely encountered in normal living. The best approach for the caregiver is to be open to what the patient desires. Patients will let you know their needs as the visit unfolds. A few guidelines are as follows:
>
> Be dependable and arrive when you are supposed to. Keep agreements and commitments. Check in with phone calls when possible. The dying are vulnerable and need to know that they can count on others. Be open and genuine; respect privacy and treat the person naturally. Relate to the person rather than the illness. Don't attempt to be the expert or express feelings that are not real. If you are nervous, say so. Sit down and establish direct eye contact if possible.
>
> Listen more than you talk, even if it means hearing things over and over again. Allow patients to talk about their illness if they desire, but don't push it. Permit ill persons to release tension through anger and resentment, even if it is directed toward you.

III. For doctors and other health care providers

Throughout this book and appendix, I have shared comments from patients about their health care providers. One could certainly write an entire book about medical professionals' communication with people with cancer, but the following comments collected from my survey speak volumes.

"I was told of my diagnosis while waiting for the results of my first baseline mammogram. After what seemed like an hour waiting in the cold sterile room in my little gown, someone who looked like Opie Taylor came and said, 'You have cancer; you'll see the surgeon tomorrow, and call your physician and she'll tell you how to cope.' He walked out, and the technician and I looked at each other with mouths open. I was stunned. I walked around the hospital for a while unable to find my car. Finally called my husband who came and got and helped me find my car, and I tried to explain to him the news. Helpful hint #1, introduce yourself before you tell someone they have cancer."

"There was a guy who tattooed me for the radiation who said he couldn't understand why people minded it. And then his hand slipped and the mark was bigger than need be. I thought he was a fool not to realize why we'd mind—a permanent reminder of a very scary time. Most people don't have to get marked up like a piece of meat."

"I liked it if the personnel doing the surgery or radiation were kind and reassuring but didn't treat me like an overly anxious person. I remember an operating room nurse who spoke to me before the final surgery and was so reassuring, just telling me her name, what would happen, that I would be able to ask questions until I went under; then, when they were doing all the things they do on the table, she kept checking in with me. It really helped to have someone there for me when everyone else was focused on the operation."

"My surgeon and plastic surgeon suggested that I have a lumpectomy and a breast reduction on the other side so I would have two symmetrical breasts. They goofed big time, leaving one breast at least a cup smaller and both with major reduction of feeling in my nipples and other areas. When I complained to the surgeon on two different occasions, he said, 'Lady, just stuff something in your bra and forget about it.' He also wanted to know why I was complaining to him and not the plastic surgeon (who was an even worse communicator). I reminded him that during more than one meeting with him prior to the surgery, he had said, 'I am in charge of this surgery so the buck stops with me.' This doctor hurt me so bad. It is so hard to trust MDs anymore. It was obvious that he thought I would sue, and my needs were very secondary to his reputation and career."

"In preparation for radiation, they do a CT scan of the chest area. Three weeks after that, I was meeting with the radiologist (whom I'd seen often in those three weeks), and he says, 'Oh, by the way, you have some spots on your liver that we saw on the CT scan.' Because I had done lots of reading about breast cancer, I knew that it metastasizes to the liver. He said, 'If I were you I wouldn't worry about it; just get it checked out.' I said, 'Why did you wait three weeks?' 'I forgot,' he said. No apology . . . nothing! Fortunately it was cysts that are not harmful, but when you are a cancer patient, news like this can be really scary, and he couldn't understand what my problem was. Even when I complained to his superiors, he refused to apologize. He hurt me badly."

"A nursing aid (the person who takes blood pressure and temperature every four hours in the hospital) told me that she looked at my chart and that she felt my diagnosis was bad. She said she had worked in the hospital a long time, and she had witnessed people die from the cancer I had. She gave me the grave stats and warned me that the chemo would be horrible. I was terrified. I didn't sleep all night and called everyone I knew to confirm or deny her stats. She was correct, unfortunately—just incredibly insensitive."

"I wanted doctors and medical personnel to recognize that I was a person—not to be my friend or anything—but to at least acknowledge that it was hard for me."

"I was forty-seven years old, and chemotherapy made me go into menopause. 'You didn't have that many years to go anyway,' my doctor said. I had a good five to six years, and I got jammed into it and it was really hard for me to deal with."

"One doctor kept emphasizing the seriousness of my condition and I wanted to scream, 'I know it's serious. It's cancer for God's sake! Can we focus on the possibility of a positive outcome?'"

IV. The Lists

The following lists are, once more, not meant to be prescriptive but are intended only as guidelines. They are culled from surveys and interviews. I cannot emphasize enough how much one patient may differ from the next; what's most important is to pay close attention to your loved one and, of course, to ask what they want and need.

21 MORE THINGS PEOPLE WITH CANCER WANT YOU TO KNOW

Again, each cancer patient is different, and there must be many hundreds of things people with cancer want those who have not received a diagnosis to know. But I've collected a few variations on similar themes to serve as reminders or conversation starters.

1. **Treat me with kid gloves, but don't let me know it.** One woman with cancer said, "Although I don't want to be treated differently (especially with pity), I do appreciate people being more sensitive to my feelings right now."

2. **I need to be touched. (Ask permission first, of course.)** A woman with lymphoma said, "Just being held made such a difference when I was sick. Just having my hand touched or my hair brushed telegraphed love and deep caring."

3. **I want to be indulged.** "Even if I'm wrong, let me be right, just for now," said someone in the throes of cancer. "Arguing is so difficult, and how much can it hurt to keep the peace when I feel like I'm at war most of the time?"

4. **I like it when you express confidence in my ability to make the right decision.** Of course this applies to everyone, but those who feel vulnerable need even more support. As Dr. Lawrence LeShan said, "Just because I'm sick, don't treat me like I'm feebleminded."

5. **I want you to help me believe in miracles.** When my cousin Billee had breast cancer, she hung a silver six-inch-wide banner across her closet door that declared in her beautifully rounded cursive, "Miracles Happen!" After she died—after the miracle of her living for seven years in spite of poor odds—that banner graced the inside of our front door for years until the print had faded almost into invisibility. Although I personally believe miracles happen whether you believe in them or not, it helps to hear from others that they believe one or more inexplicable acts of divine love might visit you too!

6. **When you say you're going to do something for me, follow through quickly.** One woman wrote to me: "I had one friend promise to come walk with me every day so I'd be sure to get exercise. She never showed up. I think seeing me bald and weak freaked her out. Another person offered to give me a ride to my doctors' appointments when I was too sick to drive myself, but every time I called her, she was too busy to give me a lift."

7. **Being sick costs a lot; offer to treat me, and maybe even insist.** Said one cancer patient, "I was really afraid about money because I wasn't working, but it was hard for me to tell my friends I couldn't afford to go out to eat. It really helped when they insisted on paying for me."

8. **I want you to be honest with me.** One person said, "I appreciated honesty. 'I don't know what to say' was something I heard a lot. Or, 'I really want to support you but don't know how. Please tell me.'" Another one said, "I was bald from chemo and sipping wine with a friend. 'Mind if I take my wig off?' I asked. He stared at my stubbly head. I prayed he wouldn't say anything hurtful. His remark was precious: 'Well, it'll take getting used to, but what the heck.' Honesty with humor is the best medicine."

9. **I don't always like to be asked about my cancer.** One man said, "The best people, for some reason, didn't make me feel awkward. They didn't want anything from me . . . no explanations, no questions. They would just make comments, which I guess if I wanted to speak about, I could, but if I didn't want to, it was okay too. They said things like, "I hope you're feeling well today . . . or I hope you're having a nice day."

10. **Don't tell me I'll be fine.** "Nobody, including the oncologist," wrote one survey respondent, "knows if a patient will be 'fine.' I know the statement is meant to encourage, but it can trivialize the seriousness of the disease."

11. **I don't want to be blamed for having cancer.** Wrote one survivor, "I think the most harmful thing ever said to me (and it was said more than once) was that I was somehow responsible for getting cancer. The idea was that if a person was responsible for getting cancer then s/he could also be responsible for getting rid of that cancer. Their idea was that cancer met some possibly unconscious need, fulfilled some childhood belief, or whatever. I found this to be an extremely harmful idea. Not only are you trying to deal with all of the stress and fear that comes with having cancer, but in addition you have to deal with the guilt that somehow, something you thought or did caused your cancer. It made me feel that the cancer was my fault, that I had somehow 'sinned' and that cancer was my punishment, that I 'deserved' the cancer because it was the consequence of my thoughts or actions. I don't believe anything else made me feel so distressed, upset, guilty, bad about myself, or hopeless."

12. **Often I want and need quiet.** "I am a writer and a performer. I can talk it up and am a very social person," wrote one woman. "When I had surgery and radiation treatment, for the first time in my life I needed silence like I need air to survive. Noise hurt my skin. I couldn't believe that I didn't want to hear words most of the time.

13. **I am unique, unlike anyone else with cancer.** Said one person, "I did not like to hear sentences that began with the phrase 'You must be . . .' I heard that a lot from people who had witnessed other people's cancer and thought that they knew what I was experiencing. They didn't know. Everybody's experience is different." Another person noted kindly, "We're not all going to be heroes; it's okay for an individual to choose her own way of coping with the disease."

14. **I don't like to hear how awful I look.** No one likes to be told they don't look good, and that's especially true for people with cancer. "Don't point out that the patient has gained or lost weight. We know by the way our clothes fit, but it is painful to hear someone mention it."

15. **I don't like to be labeled**. Again, few people like labels of any kind attached to them. But as one person with cancer wrote, "I did not like to be referred to as a 'cancer patient' or someone who is/was sick. I abhorred those labels. Even the moniker 'cancer survivor' seemed tainted with negative and long-lasting permanence. I never went to the support groups because I felt they were so mired in this identity of infirmity and suffering. That was not and is not my identity, no matter what trial I might be facing in any given moment."

16. **I will talk about my cancer if I feel the need to**. One woman wrote that it was unhelpful when people told her she should talk about it, that it would make her feel better. "I think there is a time to talk, and that it will make you feel better, but only when it's the idea of the person suffering, or when the person suggesting the talking can make the person feel like talking. Otherwise, it just makes the person suffering feel more at odds and pressured and in pain."

17. **I don't want to feel tainted or contagious**. No one does. Said one respondent, "A hurtful comment stemmed from being treated as if you're tainted somehow because the cancer diagnosis. You're a 'sick' person now. That made me feel like a brand-new inductee into the leper society of America." Said another, "People who stayed away from me as if they would catch my cancer were far from helpful."

18. **I need to have privacy**. "It is the way we choose to deal with negativity that determines the quality of our lives," noted one man. "I chose to grieve privately [for myself] and then to move on."

19. **It's hard for me to hear about your fears**. One woman wrote, "It may scare you to hear that someone you know has cancer, especially if you are young (which I was). Do what you can to keep it to yourself. The patient has enough to deal with."

20. **I need you to believe that I will live through this**. Half of the people who have cancer go on to lead long lives; they know that, but they need to know that you know that too. One cancer survivor said, "I don't think anyone can fully know what it's like without being there. I guess I would want people to know that it's not an automatic death sentence, but it is something that is always hanging over one's head, and that that is very hard."

21. **I need you to acknowledge my feelings.** This is a tough one, because although most people with cancer don't want to be treated differently, they also don't want their friends to act as if nothing at all has happened. As one woman explained: "It surprised me that some people were really unable to relate to me around the cancer at all. A few friends just seemed to disappear. Others who just didn't know how to react at all tried to pretend that I was fine. While I wasn't afraid, I did want people to know. I needed them to acknowledge me. I needed their support. So when a few close friends just seemed to pretend that nothing was really going on, that nothing was different in my life, well, that was a bit hard to take. I didn't want to have to hit anyone over the head with my situation or be overly melodramatic, but hey, what was happening to me was important!"

16 FABULOUS THINGS PEOPLE DID FOR AND SAID TO CANCER PATIENTS

As soon as they learned I had cancer, my friends and family began offering to visit, bring meals, and provide whatever kind of support I needed. I wanted my house cleaned (after all, I was expecting guests!) but was too shy to ask friends and was unwilling to ask my already-stressed husband to add that to his to-do list. Too busy and exhausted to clean it myself, I felt frightened about money and didn't think I should pay someone.

In spite of the fear, I hired Kymberli, owner of Eco-Kind Cleaning, to scour the house. After her workers completed the job, I asked Kymberli what I owed her. A cancer survivor herself, she replied, "Don't worry about it. It's on me." It rendered me speechless with gratitude.

Many who have had cancer share similar tales. Here are just a few. May they inspire you!

1. "My best friend and roommate was the reason I went in three years prior to turning forty for my mammograms. She had a lumpectomy and went through the radiation and chemo. Because of her, I had a routine mammogram in 2003 (a month before turning forty), and that's when I was diagnosed. She was there with me from the biopsy and through each and every appointment thereafter. I can't stress enough how important it is to have someone with you every step of the way.

Not only for support but also to be an extra set of ears and to think of questions you may not."

2. "I had surgery just before Thanksgiving and thought I wouldn't celebrate or [I'd simply] miss the holiday. But one friend, unsolicited, sent over a HUGE tray of Thanksgiving leftovers. I appreciated it much more than I had thought I would. I felt both included back into the world and nourished."

3. "One of my friends bought me a special gift for every treatment; my husband also treated me to special things while I was going through chemo. My family had a 'Chemo Party' for each treatment, complete with snacks, beverages, and lots of prayers and love. It made the experience bearable."

4. "I live alone and had to take six months off of work for chemotherapy. My brothers paid some of my bills, bought me a month's worth of groceries, got food for my dogs. One even gave me a gift of five thousand dollars just so I wouldn't have to worry about expenses."

5. "A good friend came over and replanted my patio pots and window box while I was hospitalized—I came home to beautiful flowers that lasted throughout my treatment."

6. "A colleague on the elevator at work asked me why I was all bandaged up and limping. He joked that I had probably overdone it over the weekend in the annual Bloomsday race—that it was too much for me. I looked him straight in the eye and said, 'I had cancer and I had surgery last week.' He didn't respond except to look sheepish. When he got off the elevator, I was left with a stranger who looked at me and said, 'You're one tough lady. Good for you! I hope it all goes well for you.' He made my day because he didn't need to say anything, but he did."

7. "One friend brought an MP3 player to the hospital, and that was fabulous because I couldn't really sleep well in the hospital and it kept me company. I could listen to music all night if I wanted to (it had about four thousand songs on it), and I didn't have to turn the light on to see it because the screen lit up. I've thanked her a million times for it."

8. "Two friends got together and brought over a cooler filled with tuna salad, egg salad, chicken salad, cut-up fruit, fresh berries, chunks of

cheese, sliced fruit bread, crackers, and nuts. I didn't ask for this; they just did it. I loved it. It was such a relief to know that I had already-prepared food just behind the refrigerator door."

9. "A friend told me that when my treatment was over, she was buying me the sexiest bra I had ever owned. We had great fun deciding what color it would be. A friend who had gone through breast cancer before me brought over her hats and other head coverings—let me know she had washed all of them and I could use them or not, whatever I wanted. No pressure. Bless her!"

10. "When I asked someone to help take down my outdoor Christmas lights in May, she came over the next day and helped me."

11. "One person sent me a thoughtful card every week I was undergoing treatment. She never missed a week. I watched the mail for those cards. (Anyone can send one card.)"

12. "The next time I know someone who is diagnosed, I would get them a gift certificate for a massage. I had never had one before in my life, and my body felt so beat up on so many different levels that the massage felt like the start of the healing process."

13. "My friends did my laundry. At the time, I lived in an apartment and had to take my laundry out. Various friends would just come collect the laundry, during the really hard stretches, and do it, fold it, and put it away. *Heaven*!"

14. "I was coming out of a meditation group, and I had a scarf over my bald head and no eyebrows. I had that chemo look. This woman looked right at me and said, 'I just want you to know I was where you are two years ago.' We talked a little. She said, 'When you go into radiation, call me if you want to talk.' It made me feel understood and hopeful."

15. "My girlfriends made it their mission every month during my treatment to schedule some kind of get-together, always with props, always designed to make me laugh and have fun. One party, they brought Groucho Marx glasses and noses that we all wore in the very swank 'W' hotel. Making fools of ourselves in nice places became our MO. Their support and encouragement in the face of what seemed an

absolutely overwhelming sense of dread was invaluable and difficult to articulate. Just writing about it makes me cry—tears of joy and of course now tears from missing that cocoon they spun around me."

16. "Two days after my diagnosis, my rabbi came over, and he sat with me, looked me in the eyes, and said, 'How are you doing?' It was really the first time someone asked me that so directly and really wanted to know. It allowed me to talk to him and to open a discussion of what I wanted to do to take charge of the situation. I felt myself reach in, find my core, and start to figure out what to do for myself to begin the healing process."

12 OUTRAGEOUS, FUNNY, OR AWFUL THINGS SAID TO PEOPLE WITH CANCER

This book is not meant to shame anyone or make people feel guilty or scared. My intention is to build compassion and provide models, and to illustrate behaviors and words that many cancer patients appreciate.

But just as important as healing words are hurtful words. In the following examples, men and women explain why the sometimes outlandish things people can say cause so much pain. Thankfully, they often cause laughter among longtime cancer survivors.

1. "Right after my mastectomy, when they took off the bandages, my husband looked at the scars and said, 'Oh, look, the Bride of Frankenstein.' I was totally devastated/hurt/angry, and if a nurse hadn't been in the room and I wasn't strung up with drains, I think I would have jumped out of the bed and strangled him. After telling him how insensitive that remark was, he said it was meant to be funny. I thought it was grounds for divorce!"

2. "When I told a coworker the first time that I had a clean bill of health, she immediately said, 'But these things come right back, you know. You need to make the most of the time you have.' It was like she was disappointed that I was fine. Lucky for me, it didn't take me long to realize she had to go [from my life], so she has no idea that I am clean and upright eighteen years later."

3. "A friend wrote me a note after my second diagnosis, saying something to the effect that she knew that I knew what a second diagnosis meant.

In fact, my doctor could not determine whether it was a new diagnosis or a recurrence so we did not know exactly what my prognosis was. I remember getting weak in the knees as I realized she was saying I would surely die of breast cancer."

4. "When I told my office staff about having been diagnosed, someone mentioned recent articles about the correlation of stress and pressure with illness—therefore of anyone in the office, she was not surprised that I was the one with cancer. (I was the executive director.) Needless to say, it made me feel responsible for getting ill, [and] that I was a workaholic, which I knew, and that somehow that set the framework for cancer."

5. "One friend actually asked me out to lunch and proceeded to tell me that she was severing our friendship because I just wasn't 'fun' anymore. I walked out."

6. "One of the most incredible things I remember is how so many 'friends' let me go. One actually told me that she couldn't handle my situation and that was that—she stopped speaking and doing things with me. I felt like a leper! Cancer is not contagious! Why are these people so ignorant!?"

7. "'You should feel lucky that your husband hasn't left you—that happens sometimes.' That was said to me by a friend in the grocery store as a 'look on the bright side' kind of comment. It was something I hadn't even considered—that suddenly I was a liability and considered undesirable as a partner."

8. "My hospital had a general list of procedures and guidelines for the mastectomy. It read to expect to be off work for approximately two weeks. Yet we are told that everybody's pain and healing process is different, and I felt the guidelines were outrageous. I was in pain for several weeks, and on top of that, had a drain tube in for almost two weeks. I was in no way ready to return to work either physically or mentally. The doctor actually got mad at me and swore the last time I asked him to extend my note one more week. His bedside manners were terrible, but I didn't want to change surgeons midstream."

9. "My mother had died just a few months prior to my own diagnosis. One person said, 'Well, you just went through this with your mom, so

at least you know the drill.' That wasn't helpful. All it did was remind me that cancer can kill."

10. "I had one friend say to me, when we were playing golf not that long after my mastectomy (since reconstructed), that she thought I was swinging the club better because there were no restrictions under my arm for swinging purposes. She thought she was being encouraging."

11. "My first surgery for ovarian cancer was a hysterectomy. I woke up in the ICU with breathing tubes. Standing at the end of my gurney was a doctor that I had never seen before. Before any of us had the chance to ask, 'Who sent you here and why?' this unnamed doctor was advising that since my family background was of Ashkenazi Jewish descent, and since I had ovarian cancer at a relatively young age, not only were the rest of my family probably going to get cancer, but 'just to be on the safe side' I *should go ahead and remove my breasts.* To imagine myself without breasts at that point was complete torture and, further, medically unnecessary. Since the surgery, I did have the genetic testing, and ovarian and breast cancer are not destined in my family!"

12. "A good friend said, 'You're so brave,' which isn't a bad thing to say necessarily, but since I actually don't feel brave (I feel scared a lot), I said to her that I wasn't feeling brave. She said something like, 'Well, I just know that if it happened to me, I would just start collecting pills,' meaning she would commit suicide. I know her mother died of cancer, and it was rough, but this was a really shocking thing to hear (especially since I've thought about suicide myself). It made me feel hopeless and depressed. She tried to make me feel better by saying, 'You've chosen life,' but that just made me wonder why I'm going through all this."

BEWARE: 26 COMMON WORDS, PHRASES, AND QUESTIONS THAT CAN STING

Many of the following items have been mentioned in the main text, accompanied by stories that illustrate why they carry so much weight. Here they are in list form, for quick reference before you visit or talk with a friend or loved one with cancer.

1. **What's your prognosis?** (Prognosis is a medical term, and it is often associated with the word "poor.")

2. **Are you in remission?** (One survey respondent said, "The term 'in remission' indicates that the cancer is lurking somewhere in your body, and it is just a matter of time as to when it will return. It makes me anxious just to hear it. I always corrected them, telling them that it was gone, period!")

3. **How is your disease progressing?** ("Progressing" denotes worsening.)

4. **So-and-so succumbed to cancer.** (No one with cancer likes to hear about others being killed by it.)

5. **(So-and-so) is terminal.** (See #4 above.)

6. **How arrrrre you?** (As Dr. Lawrence LeShan said, "If you treat me 'special' because I have cancer, you keep reminding me I have cancer. Treat me like a human being.")

7. **Are you cured?** (No one can know that for sure, but if someone believes they are, they will tell you. Asking can hurt.)

8. **When do you have to go to the doctor again?** (Let the patient bring that up. She or he may not want to think about it at the moment.)

9. **You should . . . [anything].** (Barbara Brenner is one of those brilliant women who can talk a mile a minute and make total sense. As the head of Breast Cancer Action, she understands all too well how badly people with cancer need an advocate. But that doesn't mean they need advice. She remembered what it was like when she was diagnosed in 1995. "The advice that I got—that I'm sorry I got was, 'Oh, you should get into a support group.' A lot of people said, 'If you get in a support group you'll live longer,' which is a fundamental misunderstanding of the science around support groups and what we know about support groups. There are a lot of people who are not suited for support groups. Yet people punish themselves about not getting into them because they feel that if they do they will live longer.")

10. **Cancer survivor.** (As my cousin Barbara eloquently wrote, "Cancer is in my past; I no longer choose to identify myself [as I did the first several years] as a cancer survivor. I've had many things happen in my past that I don't identify myself in terms of because they're no longer part of me, and cancer is one such thing. Eventually I think it's healthy for many people to let go of identifying themselves with having had cancer.

I believe for many it's a way to truly proceed with the new life that cancer offers each of us who have shared this experience.")

11. **It's for the best**. (As one survey respondent said, "I hated, 'This is for the best' or, 'Just think how much worse this could be.'")

12. **You're so lucky**. (One young woman wrote, "Everyone told me that I was lucky because thyroid cancer is the best kind of cancer to get since it has such a high survival rate. It sucks to be diagnosed with cancer and to have at least twenty people respond by telling you how lucky you are. I got this response from friends, relatives, doctors, alternative medicine doctors, therapists, boyfriends [and so on] from the time that I was diagnosed. It became harder and harder to hear after the first couple of months because I found out that my kind of thyroid cancer was more complicated and more insidious than most typical cases and was not over with one simple surgery or one hit of radiation. It made me feel like people didn't really care about my particular case, or how I was feeling. They wanted to feel like what was happening to me was not going to change my entire life, like it wasn't going to incapacitate me for two years, like I wasn't really going to be one of those poor people with cancer who had to face pain, fear, and mortality. I was and am one of those people. I wanted to and sometimes still want to shout from the rooftops, 'This is my experience. Look at me, not at an article you read on the Internet, not at the three other people you know through the grapevine who had my kind of cancer. Look at me and ask me what my experience is like.'")

13. **I know a friend who went right on with everything she was doing, and this was over in no time**. (Said one cancer patient, "This minimizes such a life-altering event.")

14. **You're so tough!** (Some people like to be told how strong they are, but others don't. "I hated it when people told me I was tough," one survivor wrote. "I know who I am. But this was a battle I was not prepared for. I didn't understand why it had happened to me. Even though it has now been almost six years, I still have the fear. Instead of seeing my doctor every three months, I now go every six. Each visit is stressful and I am always anxious. Fortunately, my doctor is a wonderful human being, and she understands the emotions that still play with my head.")

15. **Are you a cancer victim?** ("Victim" is another loaded term, as one woman wrote: "I am not a victim. I am one of a number of strong people.")

16. **I know how you feel.** (Even if you've had cancer, you cannot know how someone else feels. You can, however, know that you feel awful and that the person feels awful.)

17. **Pray for a miracle!** (Although most people like to be prayed for, saying that they need a miracle indicates they have a poor prognosis indeed.)

18. **You're going to be just fine.** (As Dr. Lawrence LeShan said, "Don't tell me things you don't know anything about. Don't tell me I'm going to get better, don't tell me I'm going to get worse.")

19. **You even lost your eyebrows and eyelashes!** (Saying that to a person who has undergone chemotherapy can just make them more self-conscious.)

20. After chemo: **I bet you'll be just like new in a few days!** (This can minimize what the patient is going through.)

21. Before chemo: **You'll have so much fun picking out wigs!** ("Fun" is not a word most people with cancer like to hear associated with their disease.)

22. **You're on Taxol?** (or any other drug) **That's bad stuff!** (People know chemotherapy can have awful side effects.)

23. **Just be strong and have a positive attitude.** (Again, it can be difficult, nigh impossible, to maintain a positive attitude all the time. It's best to encourage people with cancer to give themselves permission to feel whatever comes up and tell them it's normal to feel angry, depressed, or even hopeless at times.)

24. **I bet this has brought you and your family a lot closer.** (Sometimes this is true, but sometimes not. If it is not, it can draw attention to the distance and add to a patient's suffering.)

25. **Don't do that. It will wear you out.** (Few people like to be told what to do, and most know how much exertion they can take. They don't want to be infantilized.)

26. **No one knows how long we have. I could walk in front of a car and get killed today.** (This, too, can trivialize a patient's experience. Plus, getting struck by a vehicle happens quickly, allowing less time for fear and anguish. On the other hand, such a comment may show some compassion. . . .)

22 THINGS MOST PEOPLE WITH CANCER LIKE, AND WANT, TO HEAR

The words most everyone who is suffering yearns to hear are "I'm here for you and I love you no matter what." Often, what is most helpful is silence or just a "There, there. . . ." The following provide general and specific suggestions of phrases and actions that many people appreciate.

1. "I wanted to hear that people loved me, that they would be by my side through this entire ordeal, that they would do anything at all that I needed, that they would be with me even if I didn't need anything at all."

2. "Mostly I wanted to hear that they were concerned and loved me, that it mattered that I was sick, that I made a difference in their lives."

3. "I wanted and needed to hear: 'I'm going to the supermarket. Do you want to come with me, or can I pick up some items for you?'"

4. "I liked hearing, 'Can I drive you somewhere—to the drycleaners, to rent a movie?' or, 'Why don't I rent some comedies on DVD and bring them over? We can watch them together.'"

5. "It was not so much what was said, but I appreciated my friends visiting me, especially the ones from out of town. I felt their love just by them being there."

6. "I would have liked to have heard that it was normal to have feelings of depression."

7. "During chemo, I LOVED: 'I'll think about you tomorrow at ten when you get your treatment.'"

8. "Since day one I was told this by my best friend, and it helped me get through this: 'One day at a time.'"

9. "My husband said things that were comforting like. 'It's so horrible what they're doing to you.'"

10. "After my mastectomy, my surgeon came in, and the first words out of his mouth were, 'Good morning, beautiful.' It comforted me so to think that I might be beautiful even though at that moment I felt mutilated."

11. "I loved being told how much younger I looked. If they said I looked better, that wasn't as nice. Saying I looked younger told me I looked healthier."

12. "I liked to hear, 'It's okay to cry in front of me. I can take it. I can support you.'"

13. "It meant a lot to be told, 'It's normal to be terrified. I'm here.'"

14. "When people said that they probably had plenty of cancer cells roaming around their own body, and they might have some undetected tumors, too, it made me feel less alone. (I didn't want them to have cancer, but it felt good they knew we are all vulnerable.)"

15. "I loved it whenever someone left a voice mail and said, 'No need to call me back. Just thinking of you and sending love.' That's the best!"

16. "'It sounds like you're getting wonderful care from your doctor,' was very comforting."

17. "'I'm so sorry you're going through cancer treatment' is wonderful when it's said openly with a kind smile and not a pitiful look."

18. "Hearing, 'I will keep you in my thoughts—or prayers, if you prefer,' really helped."

19. "'You look so good for what you are going through,' sounded really nice to me."

20. "It felt good when someone said, 'I'm here. Let's do something fun, if you're up to it!'"

21. "It was really nice when there was no pressure, only, 'Do you want to talk about it or are you all talked out?'"

22. "It made my day when someone said, 'What's your favorite soup? I'd like to make you some!'"

20 SILLY MOVIES FOR PEOPLE WITH CANCER TO SEE

Hundreds, maybe thousands of movies can bring a smile, a laugh, and welcome distraction from pain and worry. The following list, compiled by my nieces and nephew, Amy, Sami, and Jordan and their friend Chris is a good start.

1. *Ace Ventura, Pet Detective*
2. *Airplane*
3. *Anchorman*
4. *Animal House*
5. *Being John Malkovich*
6. *The Big Liebowski*
7. *Blazing Saddles*
8. *Bowfinger*
   (one of the author's favorites)
9. *Dumb and Dumber*
   (another favorite)
10. *Duck Soup*
    (or anything by the Marx Brothers)
11. *Meet the Parents*
12. *Mr. Bean*
13. *Naked Gun*
14. *Nutty Professor*
15. *Office Space*
16. *Old School*
17. *Robin Hood: Men in Tights*
18. *Super Troopers*
19. *Wedding Singer*
20. *Zoolander*

Note: It's a good idea to screen a movie to see whether it has anything to do with illness, especially cancer, before recommending it to someone who has or has had cancer.

18 THINGS YOU CAN DO
(AFTER ASKING PERMISSION, OF COURSE)
TO HELP SOMEONE WITH CANCER

It's sometimes easier to write from the heart than speak from the heart, and greeting cards provide a great vehicle to show solicitude. Something an old friend did for me packed a powerhouse of love: At our Clayton High School reunion in St. Louis, which I could not attend because I was still recovering from surgery, Cindy circulated a poster-size greeting card for me. It included personal messages like, "I always had a crush on you" and "I pray for your peace" and "Wish you could have been here. I'm drunk," and "I hope I'll see you at our 40th reunion!" almost all signed with love.

Here are some other things you can do to make people with cancer beam.

1. Set up a prayer or silent unity group.

2. Bring animals to visit.

3. Do research for the patient.

4. Read to the patient.

5. Take the patient out for a meal.

6. Rub the patient's feet.

7. Send cards, postcards, and letters.

8. Send a list of funny movies.

9. Buy a gift of special shampoo at a beauty salon.

10. Buy or make meals or give food gift certificates.

11. Pay to have the patient's house cleaned.

12. Buy a gift certificate for a massage.

13. Buy gifts, such as plants or other things that affirm or symbolize health.

14. Do their laundry.

15. Do something for their spouse or children.

16. Take the patient to a movie.

17. Buy him an uplifting or funny book, or let him choose one himself.

18. Go to the doctor with her.

INSTEAD OF SAYING THAT, YOU MIGHT SAY THIS

Okay, so I said this wasn't going to be a prescriptive book. But sometimes we need specifics; we long to be told exactly how to say something or exactly what to do. So here are some options culled from cancer patients and survivors, health care and communications professionals, and books, articles, brochures, and websites about cancer and caregiving.

Instead of asking, "How's your health?" you might ask,

"How you doin' today?" If the answer is, "Uh, okay..." then follow up with, "I care so much about you. I want to understand how you're feeling. If you don't want to talk now, that's just fine. But I am here to listen."

Instead of asking "How did it go at the doctor's today?" you might say,

"I know you went to the doctor today. If you want to talk about it, you know I want to listen."

Instead of asking, "Why do you think you got cancer?" try asking,

"How do you think you're going to use this experience?"

Instead of asking, "Are you afraid of dying?" you could say,

"There are so many things I want to do with you."

Instead of asking, "Have you tried x, y, or z treatment?" you might offer,

"If you're interested in hearing about different treatments, let me know and I'll do some research for you."

Instead of asking, "Are you cured now?" try asserting,

"You look terrific. I hope you feel great!"

Instead of asking a question,

try saying something about your own feelings first.

Instead of saying, "I know how you feel," you could admit,

"I'll never know exactly how you feel, but I'll do my best to understand if you want to talk about it."

Instead of saying, "At least they caught it early," practice saying,

"I'm sorry you're having to go through this. I'm here for you."

Instead of saying, "Thank goodness your treatment is over and you can
    get back to normal," you might say,
  "If you feel like talking about it, I'd like to know how you're feeling now
    that you've completed treatment."

Instead of saying, "You need to think positively," try to reassure your
    friend with,
  "It's normal and healthy to think negatively sometimes. There's even a
    book called *The Positive Power of Negative Thinking!*"

Instead of offering a cliché, like, "It's all for the best," why not say,
  "No one knows why such awful things happen to good people, why all
    of us have to suffer."

Instead of saying anything,
  hold a hand, touch an arm, or offer a hug.

Instead of assuming anything,
  observe the person's posture and facial expression before you jump into
    conversation.

Instead of asking a yes or no question, like "Are you happy with your
    doctor?" try asking,
  "What do you like about your doctor?" to encourage conversation.

Instead of jumping in with another question, you might echo what the per-
    son just said. [If she says "I'm going to die, because the Iressa isn't
    working," instead of saying, "Of course you're not, you'll be fine," try,
    "It must so frightening waiting to find out if Iressa will work."]

Instead of assuming your loved one knows how much you love him,
  look him right in the eye and say, "I love you so much. You mean the
    world to me."

resources

YOU CAN FIND THOUSANDS OF BOOKS, websites, articles, magazines, films, and other resources that will help you help your loved one live with or live beyond cancer, or simply understand better what it is like to have the disease. The following list includes resources that were especially helpful to me or that come highly recommended.

BOOKS

Babcock, Elise. *When Life Becomes Precious: The Essential Guide for Patients, Loved Ones, and Friends of Those Facing Serious Illnesses.* New York: Bantam, 1997.

Berberich, F. Ralph, MD. *Hit Below the Belt: Facing Up to Prostate Cancer.* Berkeley: Celestial Arts, an imprint of Ten Speed Press, 2001.

Bolen, Jean Shinoda. *Close to the Bone: Life Threatening Illnesses and the Search for Meaning.* New York: Scribner, 1998.

Canfield, Jack. *Chicken Soup for the Surviving Soul: 101 Healing Stories About Those Who Have Survived Cancer.* Deerfield Beach, FL: HCI, 1996.

Carter, Rosalynn. *Helping Yourself Help Others: A Book for Caregivers.* New York: Three Rivers Press, 1994.

Ekman, Paul. *Emotions Revealed: Recognizing Faces and Feelings to Improve Communication and Emotional Life.* New York: Times Books, Henry Holt & Co., 2003.

Ellis, Judith, and Susan Nessim. *Cancervive: The Challenge of Life after Cancer.* New York: Houghton Mifflin Co., 1991.

Girard, Vickie. *There's No Place Like Hope: A Guide to Beating Cancer in Mind-Sized Bites.* Lynnewood, WA: Vickie Girard, 2001.

Groopman, Jerome, MD. *The Anatomy of Hope: How People Prevail in the Face of Illness.* New York: Random House, 2004.

Guilmartin, Nancy. *Healing Conversations: What to Say When You Don't Know What to Say.* San Francisco: Jossey-Bass, 2002.

Halpern, Susan P. *The Etiquette of Illness: What to Say When You Can't Find the Words.* New York: Bloomsbury, 2004.

Healy, Terry. *At Face Value: My Struggle with a Disfiguring Cancer.* 2001. To order, call 1-888-7-XLIBRIS.

Holland, Jimmie C., MD, and Sheldon Lewis. *The Human Side of Cancer: Living with Hope, Coping with Uncertainty.* New York: HarperCollins, 2000.

Kane, Jeff, MD. *How to Heal: A Guide for Caregivers.* New York: Helios Press, 2001, 2003.

Kushner, Harold. *When Bad Things Happen to Good People.* New York: Avon, 1982.

LeShan, Lawrence, PhD. *Cancer as a Turning Point: A Handbook for People with Cancer, Their Families, and Health Professionals.* New York: Penguin Books, 1989.

Ram Dass and Paul Gorman. *How Can I Help? Stories and Reflections on Service.* New York: Alfred A. Knopf, Inc., 1985.

Rosenbaum, Ernest H., MD, and Isadora Rosenbaum, MA. *Supportive Cancer Care: The Complete Guide for Patients and Their Families.* Naperville, IL: Sourcebooks, Inc., 2001.

Rossman, Martin L., MD. *Fighting Cancer from Within: How to Use the Power of Your Mind for Healing.* New York: Henry Holt & Co., 2003.

Schimmel, Selma R., with Barry Fox, PhD. *Cancer Talk: Voices of Hope and Endurance from "The Group Room," the World's Largest Cancer Support Group.* New York: Broadway Books, 1999.

Silver, Marc. *Breast Cancer Husband: How to Help Your Wife (and Yourself) through Diagnosis, Treatment, and Beyond.* New York: Rodale Books, 2004.

Sontag, Susan. *Illness as Metaphor.* New York: Farrar, Straus & Giroux, 1977.

Sourkes, Barbara M., PhD. *Armfuls of Time: The Psychosocial Experience of the Child with a Life-Threatening Illness.* Pittsburgh: University of Pittsburgh Press, 1995.

Thomas, Marlo. *The Right Words at the Right Time.* New York: Atria, a division of Simon & Schuster, 2002.

Wilber, Ken. *Grace and Grit: Spirituality and Healing in the Life and Death of Treya Killam Wilber.* New York: Shambala, 2000.

FILMS AND PLAYS

American Splendor. You can rent this movie at your video store. What I love about it is the protagonist gets cancer and lives. It's a blip on the radar screen instead of his killer. How refreshing!

Edson, Margaret. *Wit.* NewYork: Faber and Faber, Inc., 1993. This brilliant play, made into a film starring Emma Thompson, can be very frightening to patients and caregivers, but beautifully presents a realistic view of what it's like to have cancer and be objectified.

ONLINE AND TELEPHONE SUPPORT GROUPS

You can find these easily on the Internet; just go to your favorite search engine and type in "online cancer support groups." Here are just a few:

www.thewellnesscommunity.org. The Wellness Community, a national nonprofit organization, has a weekly online support group for people who have had cancer, and another group for caregivers.

www.oncochat.org. This website offers an online peer support for cancer survivors, families, and friends.

www.oncolink.com. This website, sponsored by the Abramson Cancer Center of the University of Pennsylvania, sponsors support groups. Follow the link to "coping with cancer."

www.cancercare.org. Cancer Care, a national nonprofit organization, sponsors several telephone support groups for people in all stages of cancer, as well as for caregivers. It also offers open online support groups for patients, caregivers, and the bereaved, as well as private three-month support groups.

WEBSITES, ORGANIZATIONS, CONFERENCES, AND BROADCAST MEDIA

The American Cancer Society. This organization's website is a tremendous resource. www.cancer.org

Caring Bridge. Free web pages for the ill and suffering. www.caringbridge.org.

Chemochicks. A fun and comforting place to connect with other women undergoing chemo. www.chemochicks.com

The Group Room. This nationally syndicated radio show for people with cancer airs weekly and describes itself as a live broadcast support group. The program's parent organization, Vital Options, has published a very useful book titled *Cancer Talk* (see page 252). www.vitaloptions.org

Healing Journeys. This nonprofit sponsors the free and very fulfilling and uplifting conference for cancer survivors and caregivers, "Cancer as a Turning Point." Call 800-423-9882 or visit www.healingjourneys.org.

The International Listening Association. This organization sponsors a yearly conference for professionals in the communications field but has a wonderful website for consumers as well, including a comprehensive array of listening resources. www.listen.org

Live Strong. An educational program of the Lance Armstrong Foundation. This website offers information and support to cancer survivors and caregivers so indivuduals can "live strong through the physical, emotional, and practical challenges" of survivorship. www.livestrong.org

SusanLoveMD.org. Dr. Susan Love's website is so full of information, so user-friendly and so, well, loving, that I highly recommend it. www.susanlovemd.org

MAGAZINES AND BOOKLETS

Mamm: Women, Cancer, and Community. See www.mamm.org.

Cancer & You magazine. Call 800-746-0355.

The Caregivers Handbook by Jim and Joan Boulden. Call 1-800-238-8433 or email jboulden@bouldenpublishing.com.

Coping with Cancer magazine. See www.copingmag.com, email copingmag@aol.com, or call (615) 790-2400.

Cure: Cancer Updates, Research and Education magazine. See www.curetoday.com.

Give Me Your Hand: Traditional and Practical Guidance on Visiting the Sick by Jane Handler and Kim Hertherington with Rabbi Stuart L. Kelman.

InTouch. See www.intouchlive.com or call 877-2INTOUCH.

Taking Time: Support for People with Cancer and the People Who Care about Them. NIH Publication No. 98-2059, April 1999. Call the Cancer Information Service at 1-800-4CANCER.

What's Happening to the Woman We Love? Families Coping with Breast Cancer, The Susan G. Komen Breast Cancer Foundation in collaboration with Saint Louis University. Call 1-800-462-9273 or see www.breast-cancerinfo.com.

When Someone In Your Family Has Cancer. National Cancer Institute Pamphlet No. 96-2685. Call the Cancer Information Service at 1-800-4CANCER.

OTHER RESOURCES

Ashleigh Brilliant (that is his real name!) creates lively, witty, and colorful postcards, called "Pot Shots," that I absolutely love. They are very affordable, but if you want to spend more, he has several books from which to choose. To see his work, visit www.ashleighbrilliant.com.

Comedy Cures. This national nonprofit offers support for kids and grown-ups with cancer and other diseases, and provides a free 24 hour joke line, live appearances, and other resources. See www.comedycures.org or call 1-888-HA-HA-HA-HA.

Wilber, Ken. "On Being a Support Person." *Journal of Transpersonal Psychology.* Contact atpweb@mindspring.com or call (650) 424-8764.

index